Exercise your Whole Body at Home

Wayne Lambert

Exercise your Whole Body at Home

By Wayne Lambert

Certified Personal Trainer

Certified Nutrition Specialist

Certified Life Coach

C.E.O & Founder – Whole Body Workshop

Author of Visualise the New You and Psychology of Weight Loss

ISBN 9780 9 5614 941 1

**I dedicate this book to my late grandfather
Lesley James Lambert**

Who was and still is an inspiration to me. I know he is happy
now that he is reunited with his wife, my wonderful late
Grandmother May Lambert whom we also miss so very much.

This book is also dedicated to your
Health & Fitness.

May Exercise your whole body at home provide you with
everything you desire.

Acknowledgements

As always I would like to thank my family, relatives and close friends for their continued support. My gratitude for unconditional support in whatever I do goes to Laila who continues to inspire me on a daily basis. I thank Philip Beattie a physical training advisor to the United Arab Emirate military, who gave his professional opinion on my early fitness book ideas and who is also behind the camera when we put together the home workout DVD. His steady hand, tolerance and constructive criticism were a great help. I also thank Pete Jordan the current PT advisor to the United States Marine Corps for his feedback especially during the latter stages of writing. His advice and contribution as to what the avid reader will want to see within a fitness book was much appreciated. Collectively, all of us were Royal Marine physical training instructors together in the UK, with myself and Pete specialising further as rehabilitation therapists and ex boxing champions too, we both went on to coach our respective boxing squads within the Royal Marines. Pete has recently competed in UFC (ultimate fighting) and is a training conditioning coach for many top level athletes in a variety of sports. I must not forget his wife Emma who is a personal trainer by profession, who also contributed to the book.

My utmost gratitude goes to Homrani Lotfi, a Body Builder from Tunisia. Lotfi has been a good friend and colleague of mine for 5 years or so, who is featured in all of the photos within this (first edition) book. Lotfi gave up his spare time to assist me with the completion of this book and he did so with commitment and desire. Lotfi owns his own gymnasium in Tunisia but currently works in Dubai as a fitness coach to the military. I wish him well with all his future conquests. There are a few other friends and work colleagues featured within this book who assisted me and I thank them all equally. I must pay a special tribute to Saad Zaabi, a truly inspirational physical training instructor from the United Arab Emirates. Saad is also pictured in this book who is quite possibly the most energetic trainer I have ever met. Saad always seems to be able to motivate the un-motivated and inspire whomever he meets. Saad always has good days and always shares his enthusiasm with others. His unwavering levels of energy are truly an advantage in this day and age. Saad helped me a great deal when I put together my rehabilitation book, and he is featured in all of the photos, a book that covers how to rehabilitate yourself post injury, concentrating on specific exercises to strengthen weakened muscles. Saad made it extremely easy for me by not only volunteering himself but actually enjoying the whole process aswell. He assisted me in his own time with no prompting and it was a pleasure to work with him. Apologies to anyone I may have forgotten to mention.

Table of Contents

Introduction

By opening 'Exercise Your Whole Body at Home' you have taken your first step towards achieving your physical potential and training goals. This book is loaded with the most up to date training exercises and information based on the latest scientific research. Upon reading the text, you will know how to properly, safely and effectively perform 100's of exercises and you will be ready to begin a more functionally beneficial training program whatever your aim. The true importance of this book lies with the functional exercises found throughout. Performing the exercises in 'Exercise Your Whole Body at Home' can provide significant aesthetic and functional strength benefits with an improvement in overall health and well-being as well as increased bone density, muscle, tendon and ligament strength, plus reducing the potential for injury in sports and everyday activities.

Strength training commonly uses a variety of exercises and types of equipment to target specific muscle groups and although strength training is primarily an anaerobic activity, some proponents have adapted it to provide the benefits of aerobic exercise through circuit training etc. A Fitness centre usually has a combination of free weights and machines but for those who choose the home based program you can utilise chairs, benches, balls and bands to name but a few pieces of equipment shown in the exercises in this book. Knowing what you want to achieve from the exercises you perform is a must before starting any strength program. Exercise Your Whole Body at Home provides easy to follow exercise explanations to suit your individual needs. All exercises are explained in detail so you know exactly what and where you are targeting. In all the programs the exercises we use adhere to our four rules of developing functional strength and fitness.

- Develop joint flexibility;
- Develop Tendon and ligament strength;
- Develop Core strength and stabilisers and
- Train movement's not just individual muscles.

Designing the program is the most important aspect of any strength program. In this book we have focused on whole

1

body fitness and toning whether you are an experienced sportsman looking for an edge or a beginner starting your first fitness session. In 'Exercise Your Whole Body at Home' particular attention is placed on developing functional strength and by following our principles of strength training below, your program should be designed to provide you the best available guide to physically improve your body and maximising your performance potential.

Progressive increase in load

Physiologically, training gradually increases the body's functional efficiency and in doing so the body adapts, we become stronger and fitter due to the demands placed on our body to improve its physical condition.

Variety of training methods and exercises

Training requires many hours of work with exercises and routines repeated many times. Under these conditions, boredom and monotony can become barriers. 'Exercise your whole body at Home' overcomes these barriers by incorporating variety from the many exercises provided.

Specificity for the individual

Whether you require strength, toning or increases in size 'Exercise Your Whole Body at Home' provides exercises for your individual requirements. 'Exercise Your Whole Body at Home' will enable you to gain strength to mimic everyday activities and movements used commonly in every sport. "Functional strength" is the successful basis behind gaining real strength that has lasting benefits for everyone, no matter what your goal. Many people who exercise tend to stick with what they like doing, instead of trying out new ideas but whatever level you are at the exercise choices on offer to you should be numerous. Having a variety of workouts to do and exercises to choose from can be a good thing although sometimes, variety for varieties sake can be a negative thing so just be aware that following the same program for a minimum of 6 weeks is a good guide for you to check your performance and adjust accordingly for improved results. It is good practice to test yourself frequently in order to observe your improvements. You should test yourself aerobically i.e. Walk/Jog run a set distance, record the time and try and improve over a 4-6 week period. Your local muscular endurance can also be tested for e.g. Attempt as many press ups and sit ups as you can in a set time (i.e. 2 minutes) record the amount you do and attempt to improve on that amount over a period of time. Whole body workshop offers a variety of exercise choices and templates for your ease of planning. Whether you are a total beginner or someone who needs that extra edge it will ultimately be your fine tuning and choices that will determine your results.

Chapter 1: Types of training

Below are the 3 main variables you must consider when exercising your whole body and they are without doubt the 3 most important factors you need to focus on:

1) How hard you work i.e. Intensity;
2) How many reps, sets, muscles you work i.e. volume and
3) How many times per week you train i.e. frequency

For your information:

- To achieve muscle endurance perform 13-20 reps;
- To achieve a combination of strength, size & endurance - perform 6-12 reps;
- To achieve muscle mass perform 1-5 reps and
- To simply achieve aerobic fitness perform 20+ reps

The majority of individuals who strength train perform 1-6 sets per exercise and 1-3 exercises per muscle group with adequate rest in between each set. Those who prefer circuit training have little or no rest between exercises. There are many different ways for you to strengthen your body and 'Exercise your whole body at home' has been specifically written to include the most relevant information for this edition only, this is due to it being an overwhelming subject.

In our Second Edition (Exercise your whole body anywhere) we are including advanced techniques, exercises and types of training to assist people past their plateaus and beyond. Of course we will add workouts for gym users to include fitness machine workouts and specific programs for exercises with barbell and dumbbells. If you do not use a gym at the moment then you can have all the knowledge you need prior to joining by practicing before you go (if you want to that is) but we will explain all the advantages for you within the Second Edition. The First and Second Edition books will prepare your body for great things and the content will be your personal library of knowledge to last you a lifetime.

Certain considerations need to be taken into account when planning your workout program. An individual training program could be specific to you and your needs but may not be beneficial to someone else and vice-versa. Each day that you train can be affected by how you are feeling and/or what's going on around you, therefore you will have to be slightly flexible in your day to day planning. Having a program and a plan can and will undoubtedly motivate you to achieving great results. Being prepared is the key to success and if your aim is **achievable, recordable, measurable and sustainable** then you are on the right track for permanent results, whatever your aim.

As explained before, there are many different ways you can exercise your whole body but your daily workout will generally revolve around your weekly plan, therefore if you plan to do 3 strength sessions a week then it is common to place together muscle groups For example: Day 1 - back and biceps Day 2 - chest and triceps and Day 3 - shoulders and legs. There is nothing to stop you working the whole of your body in the same session either, and in many ways the only thing that will differ is the amount of sets you complete on each body part. It is also not uncommon for people to train just one muscle group on a particular day, yet this will ultimately depend upon their training schedule i.e. Your daily, weekly, monthly plan and training goals.

Rest in between strength sessions is of equal importance and should be added to your schedule. Each person is different and therefore whether you train alone, with a partner or in a group your aim should be the same. The fact is, some people need to be motivated by others and some can motivate themselves. The location where you train will also be specific to your results i.e. do you need to join a gym, have you got your own equipment and do you want to continue to train in your own home. The fact is, you can do whatever it is that you need to do without excuses getting in the way. Your mind and your body will dictate your success whether it is daily, weekly, monthly or yearly. Whole body workshop assists you in understanding the importance of the working together of your mind and body, as one without the other is not an option for permanent success.

The following chapters include:

- ➢ Warm up, cool down and stretching;

- ➢ Different types of whole body exercises you can do and

- ➢ Specific workout templates for you to use immediately.

Chapter 2: Warm up, cool down & stretching

To prevent injuries and maximise the benefits of your workout, it is important to take the extra time to ease your body into the workout in a controlled manner. Most people know and understand the reasons why it is important to warm up, but very few even attempt or complete a warm up and if they do is it sufficient enough? To reiterate the importance of warm ups, it is best to stress that the planned workout will be more successful and you will achieve more if your warm up is adequate for what you have planned. The intensity of your preparation will ultimately be dictated by the session that you have planned.

In basic terms a warm up should involve the mobility of your joints and the circulation of blood around your major muscles. There are many pre-workout choices but generally speaking your warm up should be easy and slow yet progressive i.e. 5-10 minutes on any cardio equipment for example; the bike, rower, treadmill or anything to fire up the muscles. You can also complete the easier exercises of your program as you warm up your muscles prior to attempting the more difficult ones, depending on your plan. For example; if you are doing bodyweight exercises then an incline push up should be completed before you do a declined push up or completing an exercise with weights at 50% of your target weight.
Your warm up / cool down should also involve stretching which has the following benefits:

- Reduces the risk of injuries;
- Enhances performance;
- Helps relaxation;
- Increases flexibility and
- Reduces muscle soreness and tension.

Stretching normally involves all areas of the body, although can be as specific to the workout that you have planned i.e. only stretching your lower body prior to going for a run.
The cool down will generally include longer stretches than the warm up because the muscles will be warmer post workout, although again this will depend on your planned activity i.e. for an athlete who competes in the 100m hurdles event they will need to complete a more ballistic warm up and stretch and

will therefore require a much longer warm up phase but normally the cool down and post exercise stretches should be of a longer duration.

In our lifetime, the muscles shorten and become inflexible and even when we workout our muscles shorten due to them contracting in order to exert power. Short muscles limit our movement which can cause aches and pains and therefore stretching is very important and is an essential part of any exercise routine. There are certain guidelines to follow to ensure your stretches are effective.

- Go to the position where the stretch is felt and hold;
- Endeavour to hold each position for 10–20 seconds;
- Your breath should be slow and deep;
- You should concentrate on relaxing;
- You should ensure good form and posture;
- You should always stretch warm muscles not cold;
- You should always avoid bouncing movements and
- You should always be patient.

Regular stretching will of course improve your flexibility, more importantly though it will assist in improving your performance

Overleaf, we have included many stretches for you and the choices included are some of the most common and easiest stretches to perform and to that end the variations included are by no means exhaustive. You should include the stretches that work best for you within your daily workouts. If time is limited then you can include stretching during your workout to save time

STRETCHING

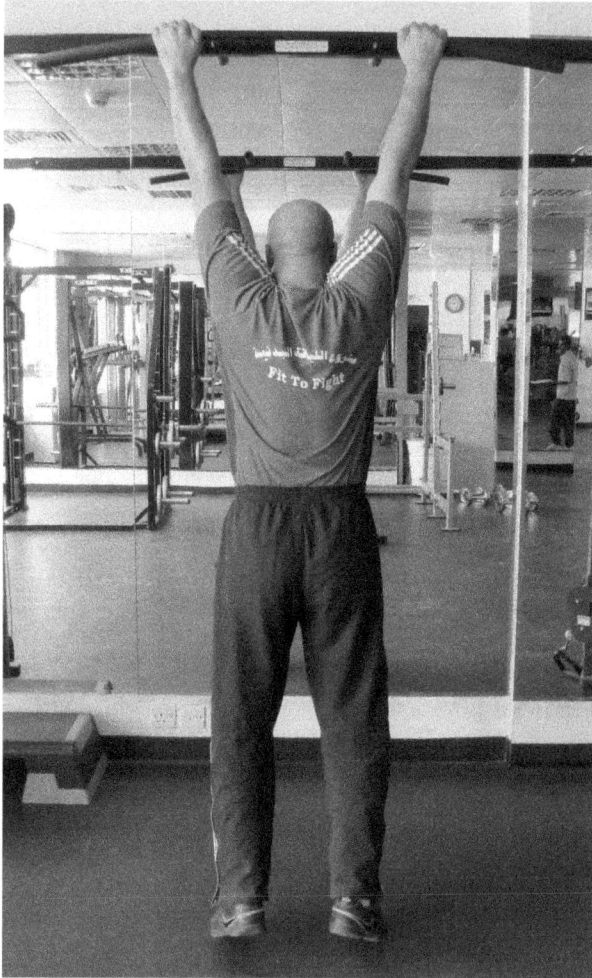

Your Whole Body

Back

Exercise 1.1 – Forward bend (supported)

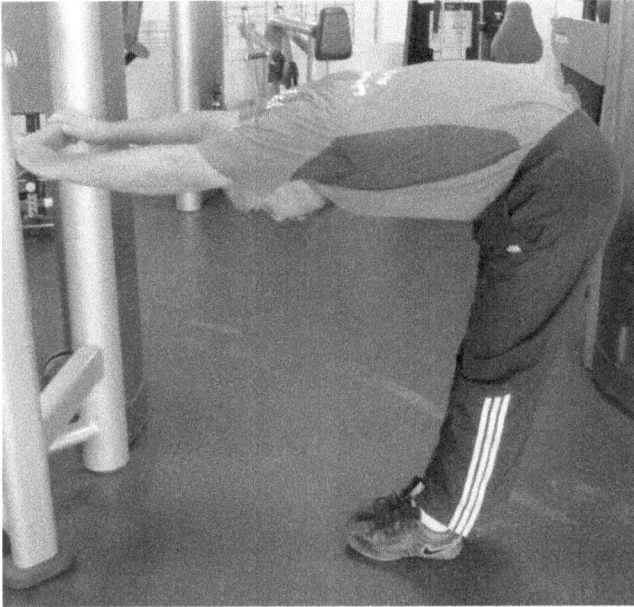

EXERCISE DESCRIPTION

Choose a solid object that is around chest height and from the standing straight position ensure that your feet are flat on the floor and shoulder width apart. Place your hands on the object, bend your knees and under control lean forwards by bending at the waist. You should feel a stretch on the lower back as you hold the position, your breathing should be controlled at all times. Return slowly to the start position and repeat accordingly.

Exercise 1.2 – Forward bend (un-supported)

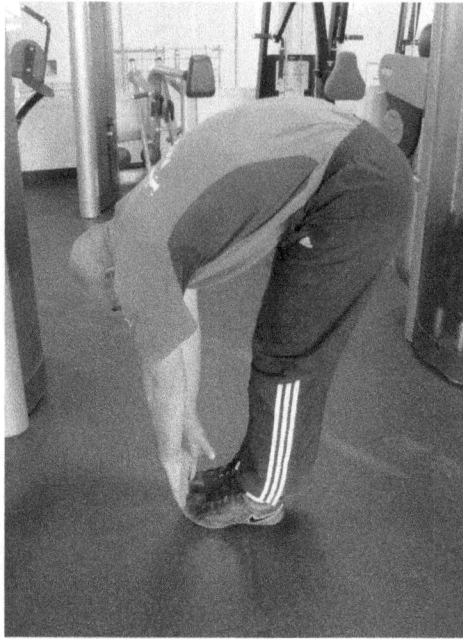

EXERCISE DESCRIPTION

From the standing straight position ensure that your feet are flat on the floor and wide enough apart that you have enough balance. Bend your knees and under control lean forwards and attempt to touch your toes by bending at the waist. You should feel a stretch on the lower back and hamstrings (back of the legs) as you hold the position, your breathing should be controlled at all times. Make a mental note of how far you have reached down and attempt to get lower each time without straining yourself. Return slowly to the start position and repeat accordingly.

Exercise 1.3 – Forward bend (assisted)

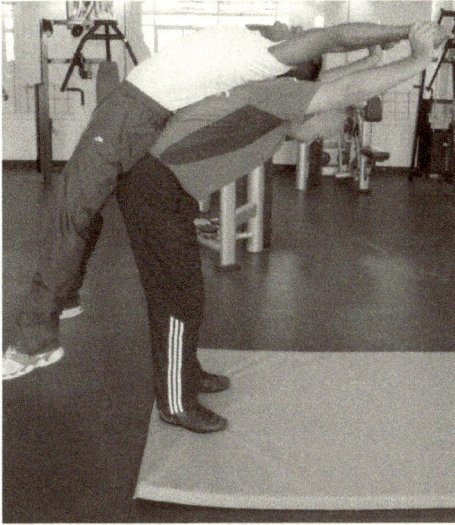

EXERCISE DESCRIPTION

It is important to note that this stretch should be done with extreme care & caution! Choose a person that is fairly light and around the same height as you and from the standing straight position ensure that your feet are flat on the floor and shoulder width apart with your knees bent. Place your partner's hands in yours, bend your knees, tense your abdominals and under immense control lean forwards by bending at the waist. You should feel a stretch on the lower back as you hold the position, your breathing should be controlled at all times. Return slowly to the start position and repeat accordingly.

Exercise 1.4 – Tree hug

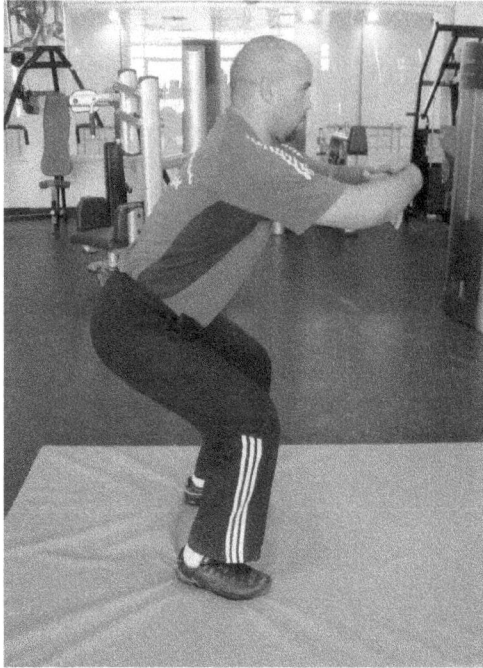

EXERCISE DESCRIPTION

From the standing straight position ensure that your feet are flat on the floor and wide enough apart that you have enough balance. Bend your knees and under control lean forwards slightly and act as though you are hugging a large tree which will round off your back and give you a good stretch around the upper to mid section of the back. Hold your abdominals in whilst controlling your breathing at all times. Return slowly to the start position and repeat accordingly.

Exercise 1.5 – Twist & hold

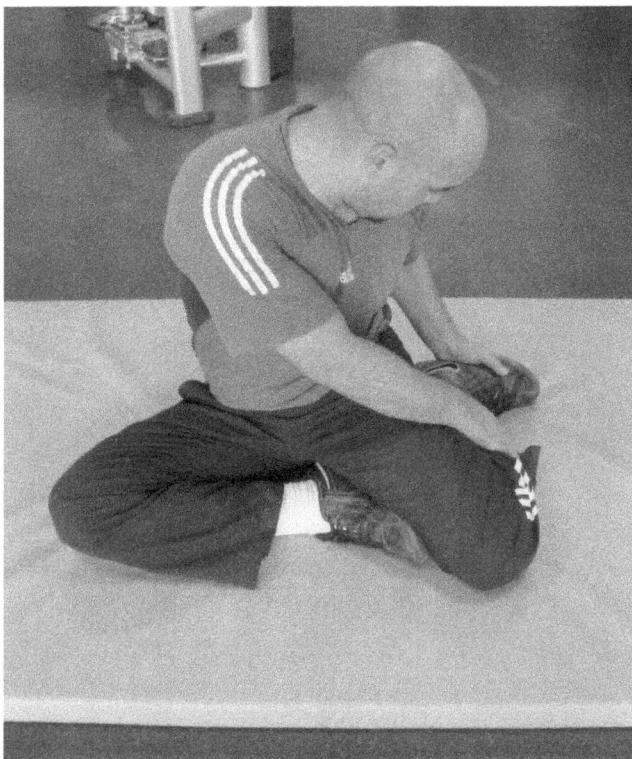

EXERCISE DESCRIPTION

From the kneeling position twist to one side as far as you can go whilst breathing out without straining yourself. Breathe in as you return to the centre and repeat to the opposite side. This will stretch out your obliques at the side of your body but will also stretch out the lats and muscles positioned around the lower back. To make it easier you can try it whilst seated in a chair.

Exercise 1.6 – Pelvic tilt

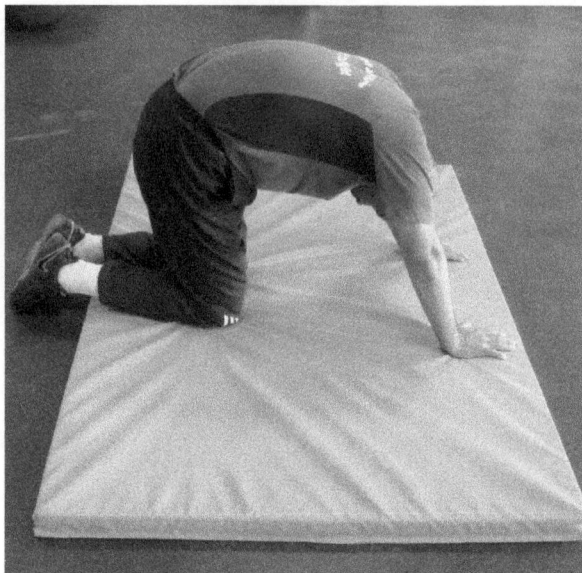

EXERCISE DESCRIPTION

From the kneeling position ensure that your hands are level with your shoulders and your knees and hands are in line as much as possible. Your shoulders should be relaxed and your hips and shoulders initially should remain facing towards the ground along with your head and eyes. Initiate the movement from the abdominals and tilt your pelvis to the rear as you breathe out whilst pulling your head inwards. Slowly return to the start position whilst breathing in, repeat the movement in a controlled manner. Maintaining control throughout the movement is key whilst breathing correctly.

Exercise 1.7 – Knees to chest

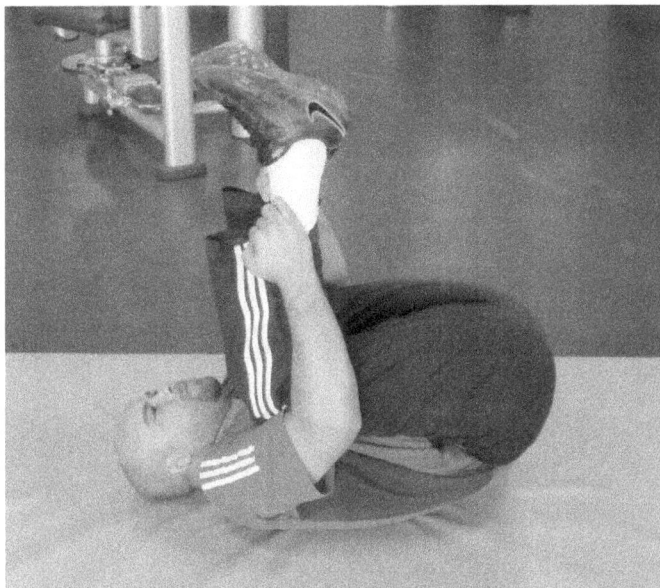

EXERCISE DESCRIPTION

From the back lying position ensure that your hips and shoulders are facing upwards along with your head and eyes. Reach forwards to grasp the back of your legs and roll backwards until your back is flat on the floor. Maintain this hold as you feel the stretch which combines the hamstrings, glutes and lower back. Return to the start position and repeat.

Chest

Exercise 2.1 – Hands to rear

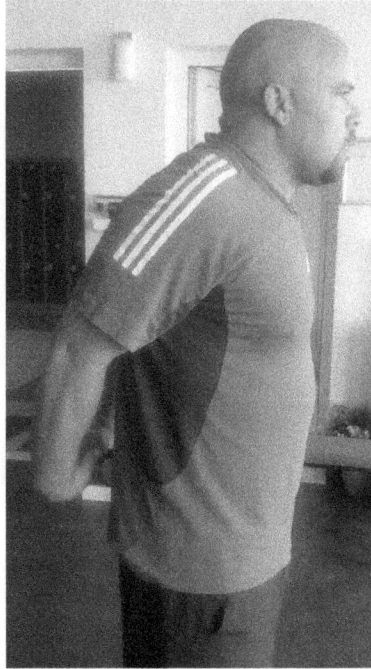

EXERCISE DESCRIPTION

Stand upright with your hands clasped together behind your back, pull your arms as far from your body as possible whilst at the same time pulling your shoulders back and sticking your chest out. Your shoulders should be relaxed with minimum tension with your head and eyes facing forwards, breathe normally.

Exercise 2.2 – Wall Stretch 1

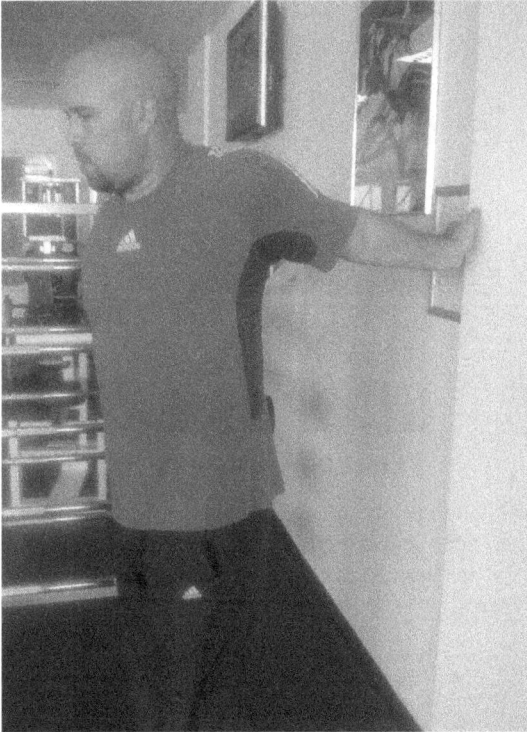

EXERCISE DESCRIPTION

Stand upright and place one hand on a wall just below shoulder height, turn your body away from the wall whilst sticking your chest out. Your arm should be straight at all times with your shoulders relaxed, breathe normally.

Exercise 2.3 – Wall Stretches 2 & 3

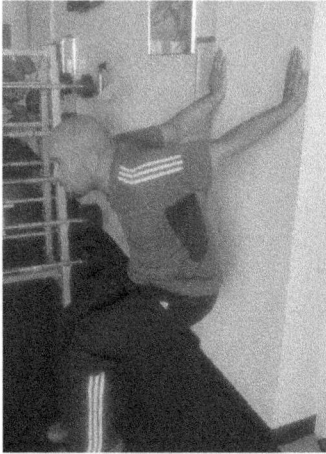

EXERCISE DESCRIPTION

Initially, stand upright and place both hands on a wall just below shoulder height, bend at the waist as your body weight allows for the straight arms to apply maximum stretch on the chest. Your shoulders should be relaxed as you breathe normally.

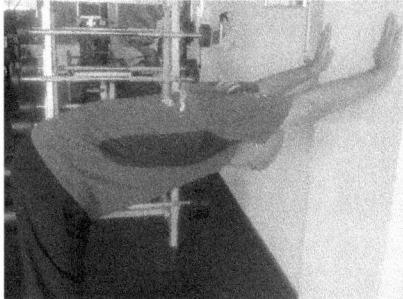

Exercise 2.4 – Arms above head (floor stretch)

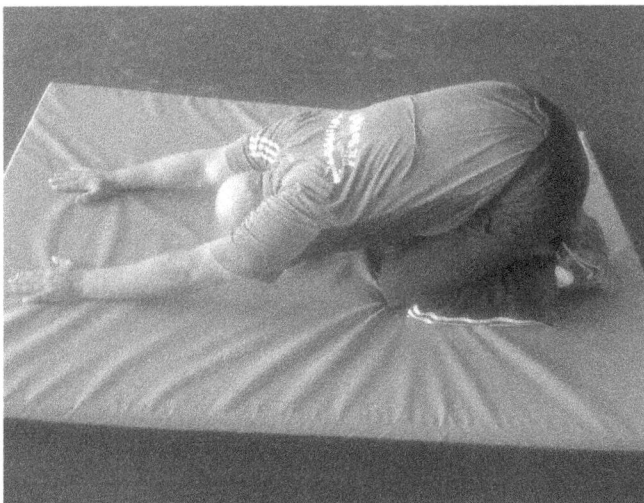

EXERCISE DESCRIPTION

Kneel on all fours and lean forwards onto the mat with your arms outstretched in front of you; allow your bodyweight to apply a maximum stretch on the chest. Your shoulders should be relaxed as you breathe normally.

Exercise 2.5 – Arm out to side (floor stretch)

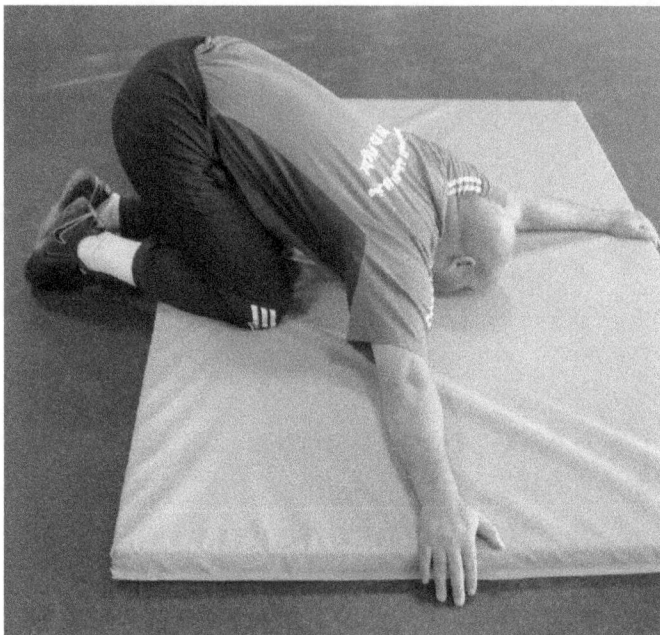

EXERCISE DESCRIPTION

Kneel on all fours and lean forwards onto the mat with one arm outstretched to the side; allow your bodyweight to apply a maximum stretch on the chest. Your arm should be shoulder height and as relaxed as possible as you breathe normally.

Shoulders

Exercise 3.1 – Most Common Deltoid Stretch

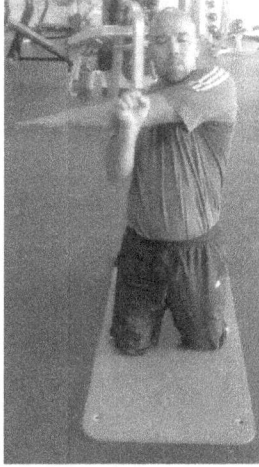

EXERCISE DESCRIPTION

Kneel on all fours or stand upright and place your arm across your body whilst pulling it in with the opposite arm, this stretch can be increased further by another person assisting.

Breathe naturally

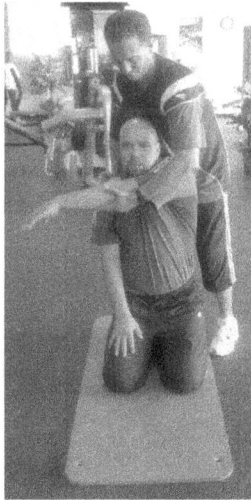

Exercise 3.2 – Anterior Deltoid Stretch

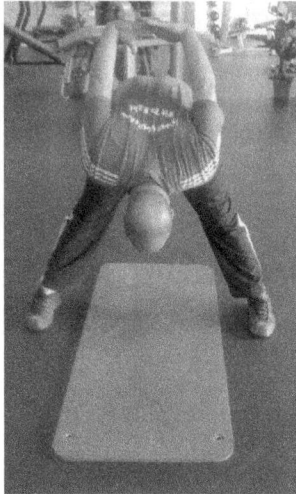

EXERCISE DESCRIPTION

Kneel on all fours or stand upright and place your arms behind you whilst pushing them close together, this stretch can be increased further by bending forward or having another person assist you.

Breathe naturally

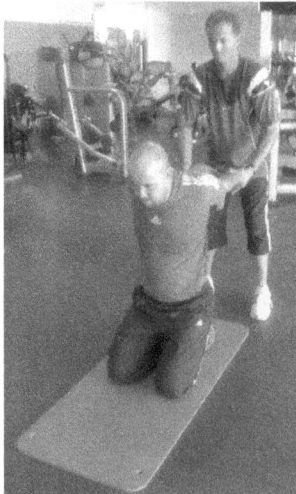

Exercise 3.3 – Posterior Deltoid Stretch

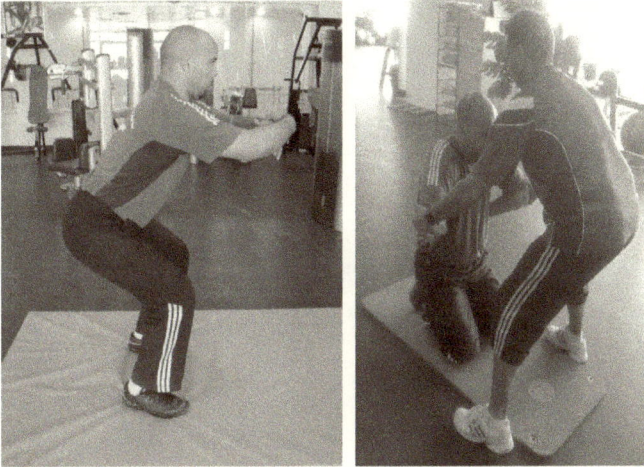

EXERCISE DESCRIPTION

From the standing straight position ensure that your feet are flat on the floor and wide enough apart that you have enough balance. Bend your knees and under control lean forwards slightly and act as though you are hugging a large tree which will round off your back and give you a good stretch around the upper to mid section of the back. Hold your abdominals in whilst controlling your breathing at all times Return slowly to the start position and repeat accordingly. This stretch can be increased further by having another person assist you, whether you are standing or kneeling place your hands behind you whilst pushing your elbows to the front of you. Breathe naturally

Exercise 3.4 – Additional Deltoid Stretches (Both arms)

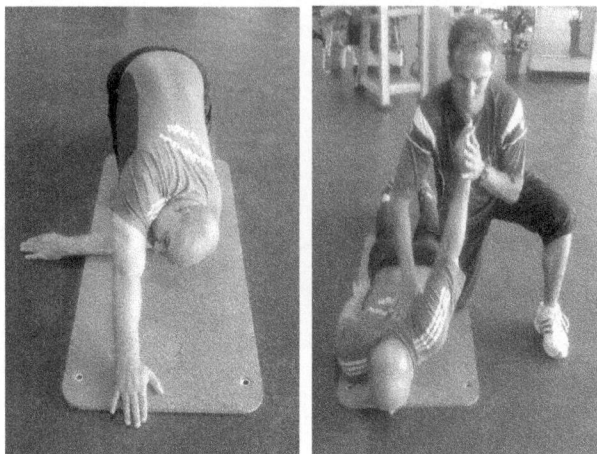

EXERCISE DESCRIPTION

All of the stretches shown are a variation of all the stretches already covered, whether you are standing, kneeling, lying down, alone or assisted the principles still apply. So long as you hold the correct position, breathe naturally and maintain good posture and form to everything you do.

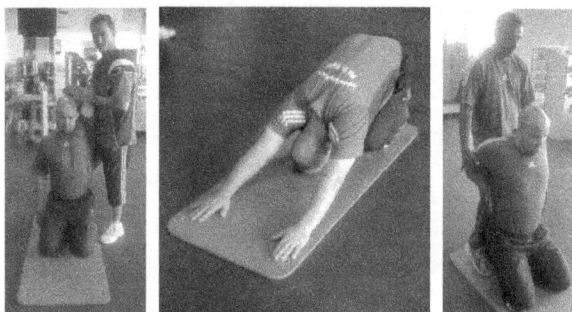

Biceps

Exercise 4.1 – Common Bicep stretch

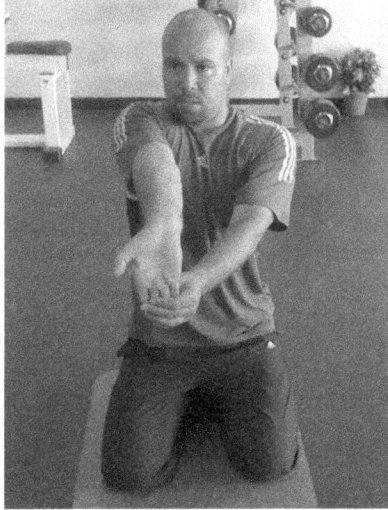

EXERCISE DESCRIPTION

Pull your wrist backwards and away from your forearm whilst
ensuring that your arm is straight, attempt to lock your elbow
out in a safe manner.

Exercise 4.2 – Kneeling (all fours) stretch

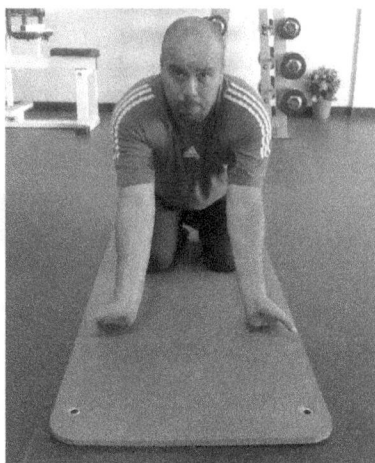

EXERCISE DESCRIPTION

Kneel on the floor and place your arms out in front of you with the forearms facing away from you. Your hands should be facing towards you and you should ensure that your arms are straight, attempt to lock your elbow out in a safe manner. Roll your bodyweight forward of your hands to increase the stretch further but be careful as your wrists are delicate joints.

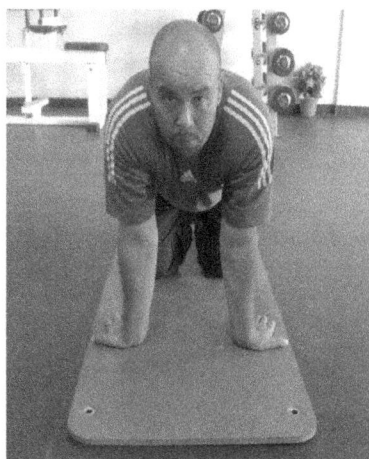

Exercise 4.3 – Arm out to side (floor stretch)

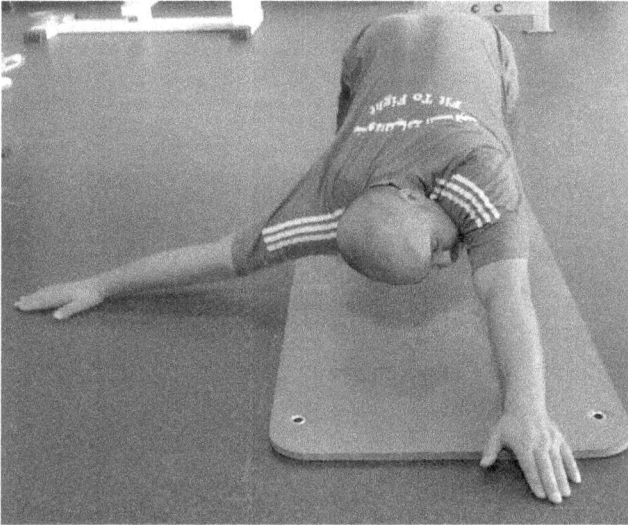

EXERCISE DESCRIPTION

Kneel on all fours and lean forwards onto the mat with one
arm outstretched to the side and one out to the front; allow
your bodyweight to apply a maximum stretch on the bicep.
Your arm should be shoulder height and straight but as relaxed
as possible as you breathe normally.

Exercise 4.4 – Seated (arms to rear) stretch

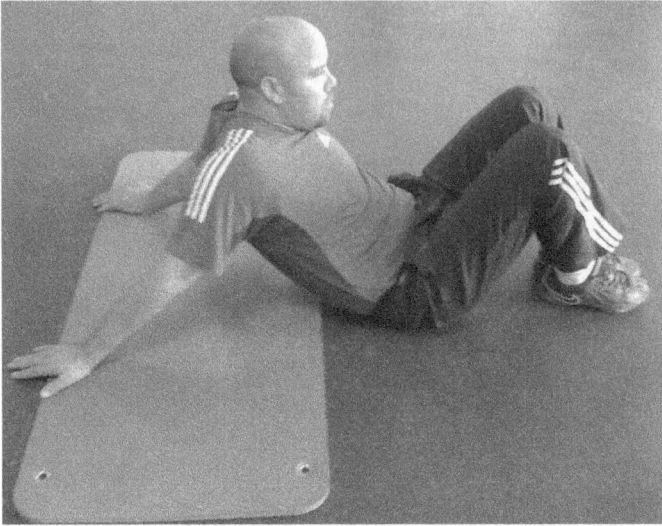

EXERCISE DESCRIPTION

Sit on the floor with your arms behind you, your arms should be completely straight with your shoulders relaxed. Use your upper bodyweight to apply a greater stretch on the biceps and safely ensure that your wrists are bent with your hands facing away from your forearms at all times.

Triceps

Exercise 5.1 – Most common triceps stretch

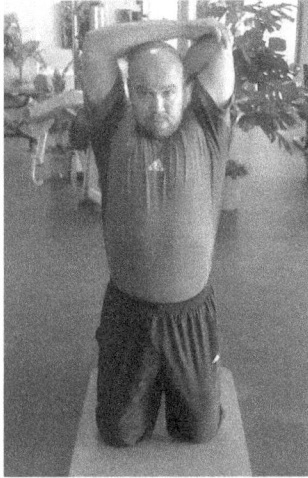

EXERCISE DESCRIPTION

Start in the kneeling position with your hips, shoulders head and eyes inline and facing forwards. Place one arm behind your head and fully bend it at the elbow, attempt to place your hand as far down the centre of the back as possible. Increase the stretch by applying a resistance with the opposite arm, breathe normally.

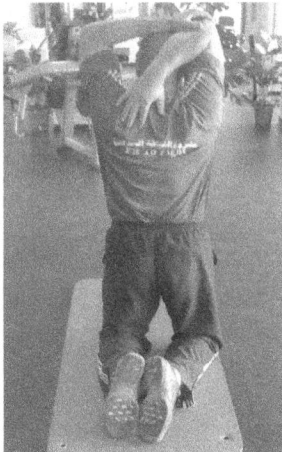

Exercise 5.2 – Assisted using a towel

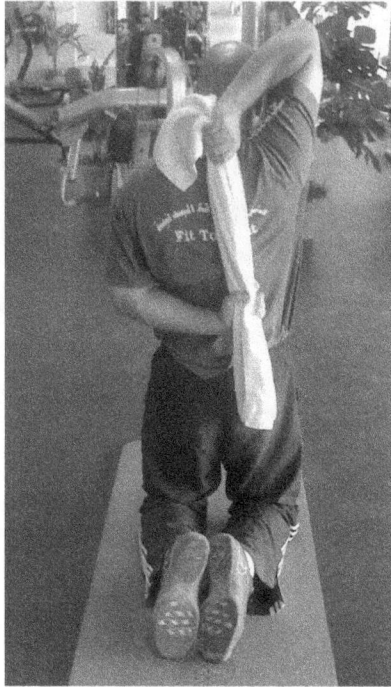

EXERCISE DESCRIPTION

Start in the kneeling position with your hips, shoulders, head
and eyes inline and facing forwards. Place a towel in one hand
and place it behind your head, this arm should be fully bent at
the elbow. With your opposite hand pull the towel down
which should in turn increase the stretch of the arm you are
stretching, breathe normally

Exercise 5.3 – Assisted using a bench

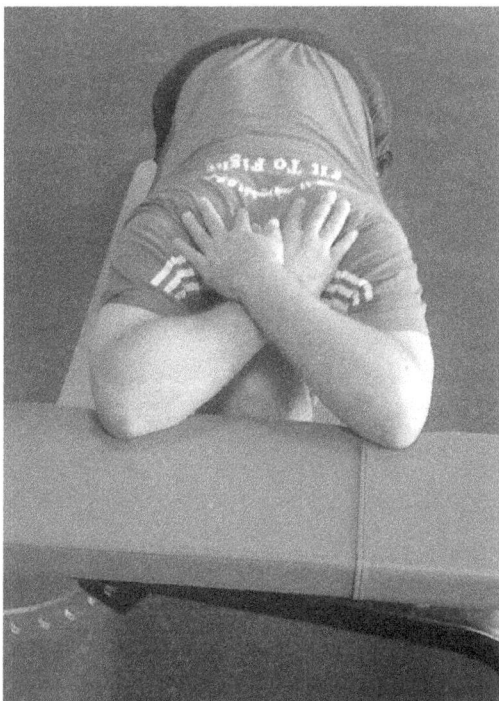

EXERCISE DESCRIPTION

Start in the kneeling position, your hands crossed above your head and down the centre of your back, place your elbows on a flat sturdy surface. Use your bodyweight to move your hands as far down the centre of the back as possible. Increase the stretch by leaning more forward using your elbows down onto the bench, breathe normally

Exercise 5.4 – Assisted using a partner

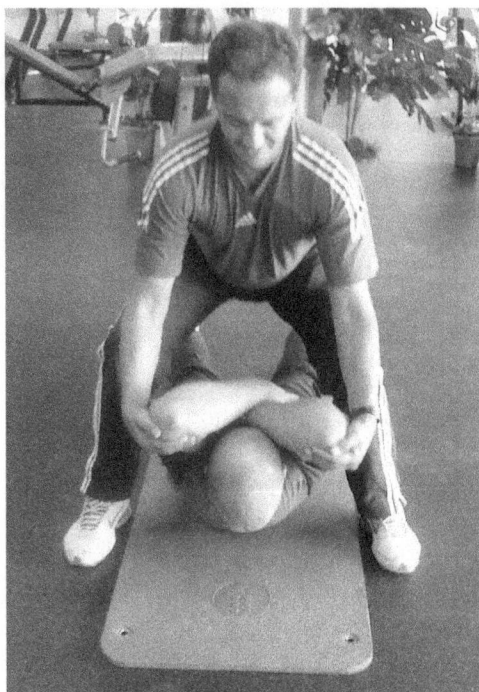

EXERCISE DESCRIPTION

Start in the front lying position, your hands crossed above your head and down the centre of your back, your partner should hold your elbows pull you off the floor and attempt to move your hands as far down the centre of the back as possible by pushing your elbows down under control. Your partner should have a wide stance and keep his/her back straight, breathe normally

Exercise 5.5 – Variations

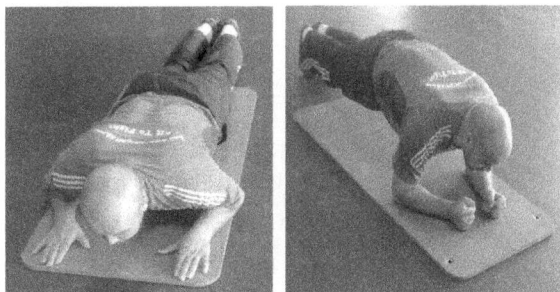

EXERCISE DESCRIPTION

All of the triceps stretches require your arms to be fully bent at the elbow whether they are behind your head or in front of you. Utilizing a partner (safely) can greatly increase your stretching abilities, holding a position (isometric – top right) can also provide a stretch so long as you maintain good form and good posture and breathe normally.

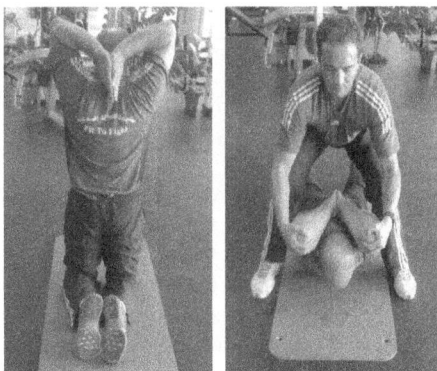

Legs

Exercise 6.1 – Hip flexors

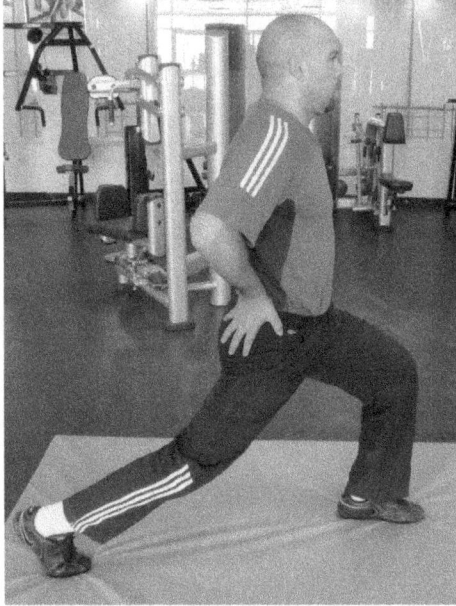

EXERCISE DESCRIPTION

Stand upright with your feet flat on the floor and your head, eyes, hips and shoulders inline and facing forwards. Take a step backwards and endeavour to keep your body inline as mentioned above. To get a good stretch you must push your hips forwards whilst leaning backwards with the upper body, therefore stretching your hip flexors at the top of the upper thigh of each leg. Breathe under control and repeat with the opposite leg.

Exercise 6.2 – Glutes

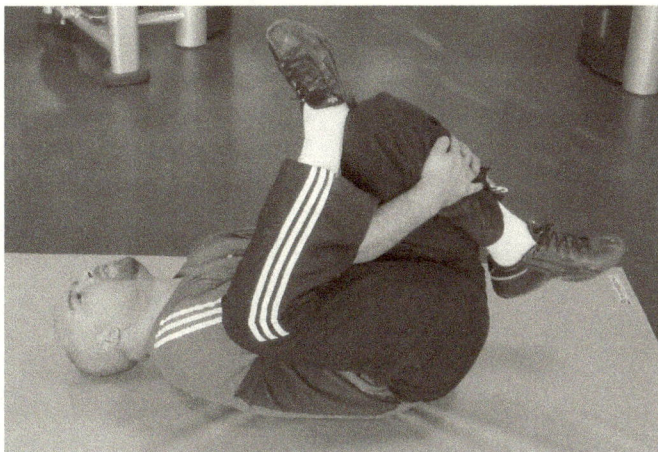

EXERCISE DESCRIPTION

Lie on your back with your head, eyes, hips and shoulders inline and facing forwards. Place your hands around the sides of the leg that you are stretching, grasp your shin, pull the leg towards your chest and rock backwards. This stretch is for your glutes and you can do the same stretch standing up on one leg with the other leg crossed over the other in the same position as the picture although this requires more balance from the standing leg and you have to squat down to increase the stretch further. Breathe under control and repeat with the opposite leg.

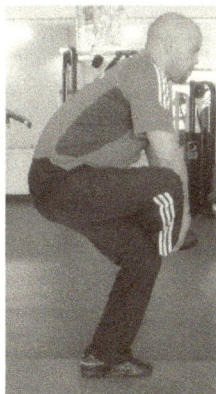

Exercise 6.3 – Hamstrings

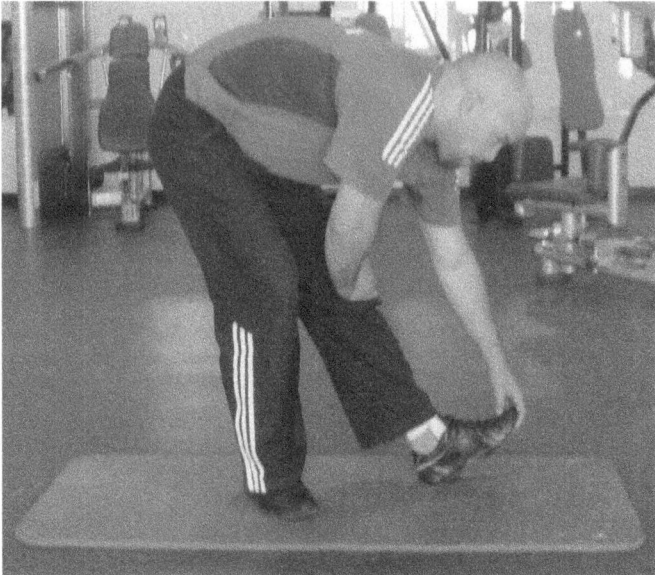

EXERCISE DESCRIPTION

Stand upright with your feet flat on the floor and your head, eyes, hips and shoulders inline and facing forwards. Take a step forward with one leg and bend at the hips (forwards and down) towards your toe as far as you can safely go. To get a good stretch you can raise the toe off the ground. Breathe under control and repeat with the opposite leg.

Exercise 6.4 – Quadriceps

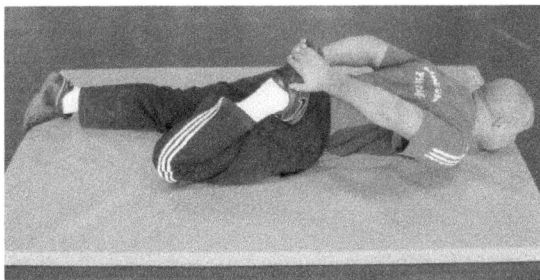

EXERCISE DESCRIPTION

Lie on your front with your head, eyes, hips and shoulders inline and facing forwards. Bend one leg towards your backside and place your hands around the foot grasping it securely. This stretch is for your quadriceps and you can do the same stretch standing up on one leg with the other leg bent behind you in the same position as the picture although this requires more balance from the standing leg. To increase the stretch further you must push your hips forwards and pull the foot in more, you can also stretch both legs together. Breathe under control and repeat with the opposite leg.

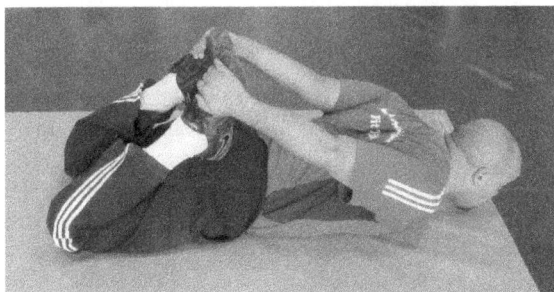

Exercise 6.5 – ITB

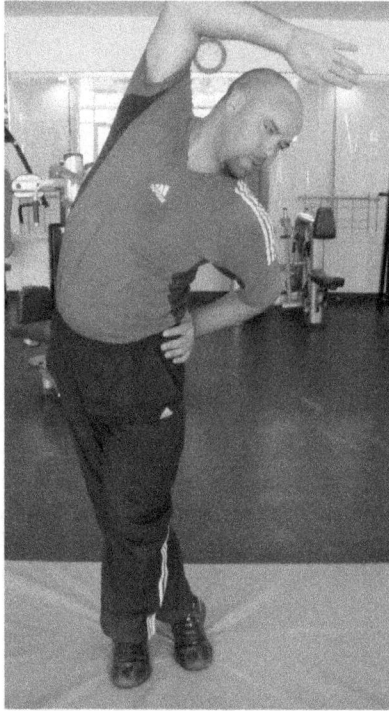

EXERCISE DESCRIPTION

Stand upright with your feet flat on the floor and your head, eyes, hips and shoulders inline and facing forwards. Place one leg behind the other and lean with your upper body in the opposite direction i.e. If you place your right leg behind then you must lean left, pushing your hips right. To get a better stretch you can lean over further with your upper body. Breathe under control and repeat with the opposite leg.

Exercise 6.6 – Inner thigh

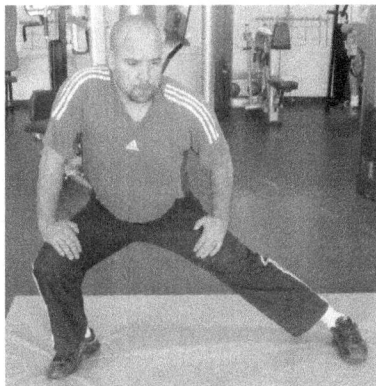

(A)

EXERCISE DESCRIPTION

With your head, eyes, hips and shoulders inline and facing forwards, ensure that whichever stretch you are doing for the inner thigh that you adjust your bodyweight accordingly to get the maximum stretch from the relevant muscles. Breathe under control and repeat with the opposite leg. For stretch (A) the leg that you are stretching should be straight with your upper bodyweight forward of your hips whilst pushing the straight leg downwards. For stretch (B) the legs should be bent and the knees pushed outwards with the elbows ensuring that the feet are together and facing each other, again your upper bodyweight should be forward of your hips.

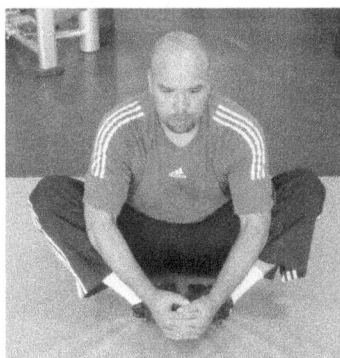

(B)

Exercise 6.7 – Calf

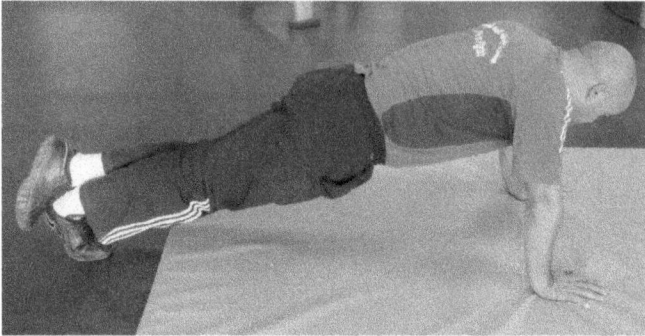

EXERCISE DESCRIPTION

With both your hands and legs resting on the floor, ensure that your head, eyes, hips and shoulders inline and facing forwards. Place one leg on top of the other whilst pushing the heel of the leg that you are stretching as close to the floor as you can in a safe and controlled manner. Breathe under control and repeat with the opposite leg. You can achieve the same stretch in the standing position, just keep your heels lower than your toes.

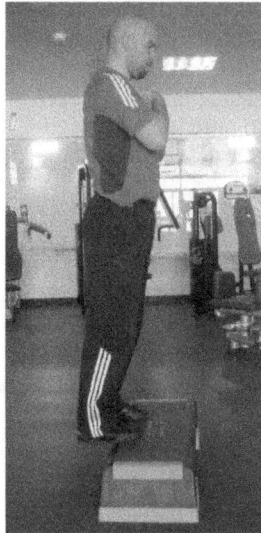

Flexibility program – (template)

Timings will depend on whether it is a warm up or cool down.

Back stretches	Time	Sets	Remarks
Forward bends			
Tree hug			
Twist & hold			
Pelvic tilt			
Knees to chest			
Chest stretches	**Time**	**Sets**	**Remarks**
Hands to rear			
Wall Stretch 1			
Wall Stretches 2 & 3			
Arms above head			
Arm out to side-floor			
Shoulder stretches	**Time**	**Sets**	**Remarks**
Most Common			
Anterior Deltoid			
Posterior Deltoid			
Additional			
Bicep stretches	**Time**	**Sets**	**Remarks**
Common stretch			
Kneeling (all fours)			
Arm out to side-floor			
Seated (arms to rear)			
Triceps stretches	**Time**	**Sets**	**Remarks**
Common stretch			
Using a towel			
Using a bench			
Using a partner			
Variations			
Leg stretches	**Time**	**Sets**	**Remarks**
Hip flexors			
Glutes			
Hamstrings			
Quadriceps			
ITB			
Inner thigh			
Calf			

BODYWEIGHT
EXERCISES

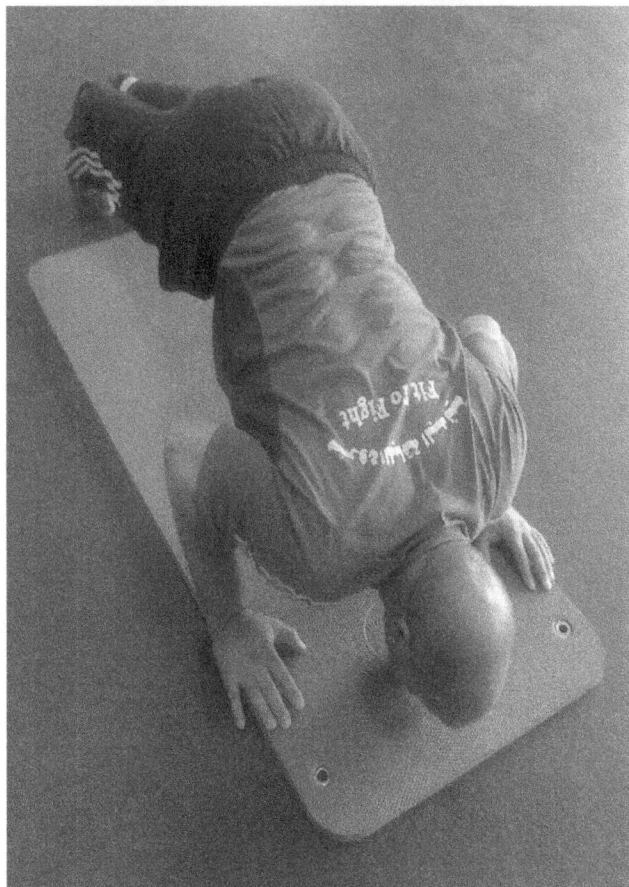

Chapter 3

Back

Exercise 1.1 – Seated back extension

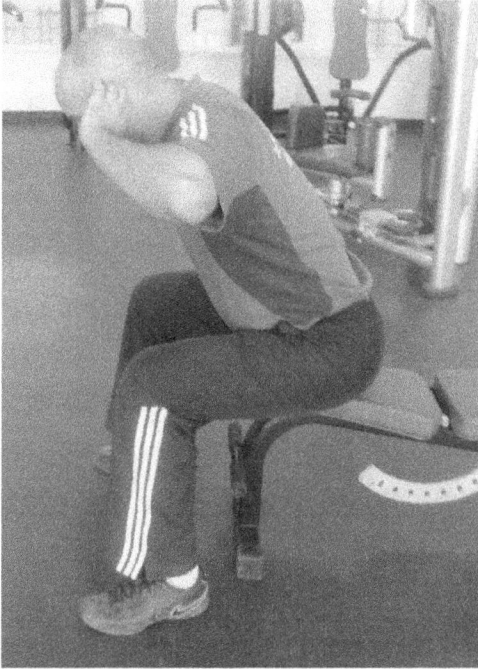

EXERCISE DESCRIPTION

From the seated position ensure that your feet are flat on the floor and that your hips, shoulders, head and eyes are inline. Lean forwards under the control of your abdominals whilst breathing in, under control move your upper body backwards contracting the lower back muscles whilst breathing out. Repeat the movement in a controlled manner.

Exercise 1.2 – Standing back extension

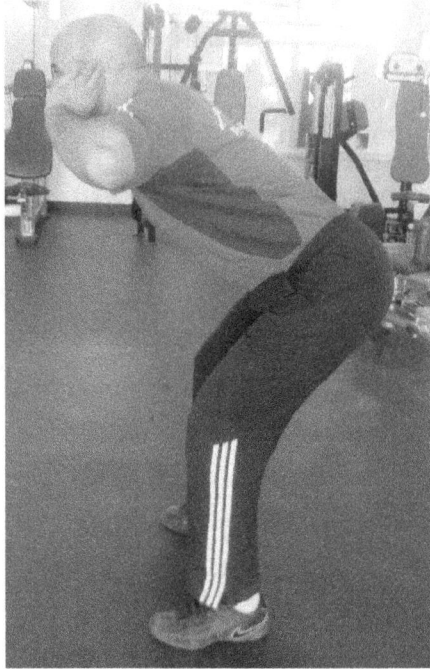

EXERCISE DESCRIPTION

From the standing position ensure that your feet are shoulder width apart and flat on the floor and that your hips, shoulders, head and eyes are inline. Lean forwards under the control of your abdominals whilst breathing in, under control move your upper body backwards contracting the lower back muscles whilst breathing out. Repeat the movement in a controlled manner.

Exercise 1.3 – Alternate arm & leg raise 1

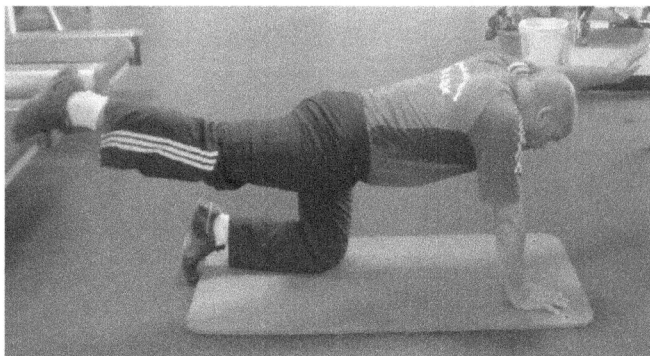

EXERCISE DESCRIPTION

From the kneeling position ensure that your hands are level with your shoulders and your knees and hands are in line. Your shoulders should be relaxed and your hips and shoulders should remain facing towards the ground along with your head and eyes. Initiate the movement from the abdominals and raise one arm and the opposite leg simultaneously whilst looking forwards as you breathe out. Hold the position as if you are balancing something on your back and slowly return to the start position whilst breathing in. Repeat the movement with the opposite arm and leg in a controlled manner. If this is too difficult you can begin by moving one arm or one leg only and then progress accordingly. Maintaining control throughout the movement is key whilst breathing correctly.

Exercise 1.4 – Alternate arm & leg raise 2

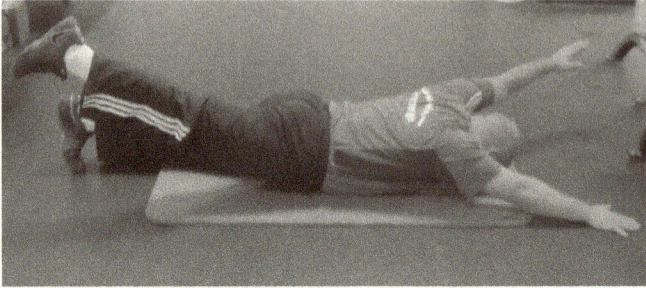

EXERCISE DESCRIPTION

From the lying position ensure that your shoulders are relaxed and your hips and shoulders remain facing towards the ground along with your head and eyes. Initiate the movement from the abdominals and raise one arm and the opposite leg simultaneously whilst looking forwards as you breathe out. Hold the position as if you are balancing something on your back and slowly return to the start position whilst breathing in. Repeat the movement with the opposite arm and leg in a controlled manner. If this is too difficult you can begin by moving one arm or one leg only, then both arms only and then both legs only. You can then progress accordingly as explained above. Maintaining control throughout the movement is the key whilst breathing correctly.

Exercise 1.5 – Straight leg hold

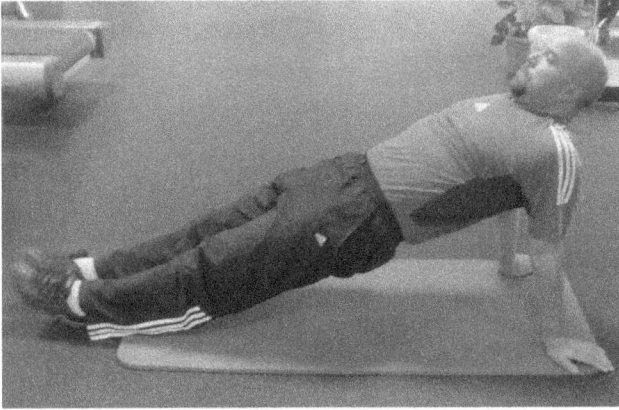

EXERCISE DESCRIPTION

Start off by sitting on the floor with your legs outstretched, place your hands level with your shoulders and ensure and that your hips, shoulders, head and eyes are inline. Ensuring that your hands are flat on the floor, support your bodyweight as you raise your hips off the ground whilst breathing out. Hold the position as you contract both your abdominals and lower back, return to the start position under control whilst breathing in. Repeat the movement accordingly

Exercise 1.6 – Plank progressions

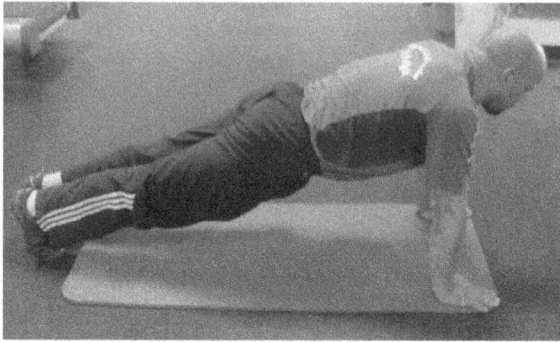

EXERCISE DESCRIPTION

From the kneeling position ensure that your hands are level with your shoulders and your knees and hands are in line. Your shoulders should be relaxed and your hips and shoulders should remain facing towards the ground along with your head and eyes. Initiate the movement from the abdominals and move your legs to the rear whilst looking forwards as you breathe out. Hold the position as if you are balancing something on your back and breathe in and out in a controlled manner. Hold the position for as long as possible but you should aim to work towards 2 minutes. As you tire concentrate on your breathing whilst compressing your abdominals and lower back, tense your whole body (not shoulders) to assist you in keeping good form. If you need to rest, slowly return to the start position and repeat the movement in a controlled manner. If this is too difficult you can begin by placing your hands on a raised (secure) platform and do the same as above. You can make it more difficult by doing the same movement but on your forearms ensuring your elbows are level with your shoulders and also progress by placing your legs on a raised (secure) platform. Maintaining control throughout the movement is important whilst breathing correctly.

Exercise 1.7 – Hip raises

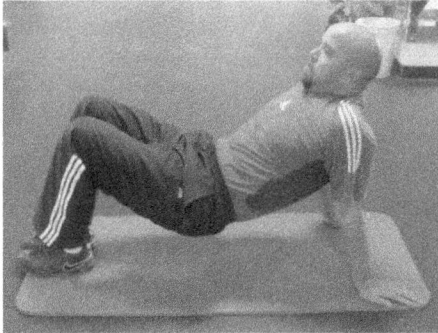

EXERCISE DESCRIPTION

Start off by sitting on the floor with your knees bent and feet flat on the floor, place your hands level with your shoulders and ensure your hips and shoulders are facing forwards along with your head and eyes. Ensuring that your hands are flat on the floor, support your bodyweight as you raise your hips off the ground whilst breathing out. Hold the position as you contract your abdominals lower back and Glutes. Return to the start position under control whilst breathing in, repeat the movement accordingly.

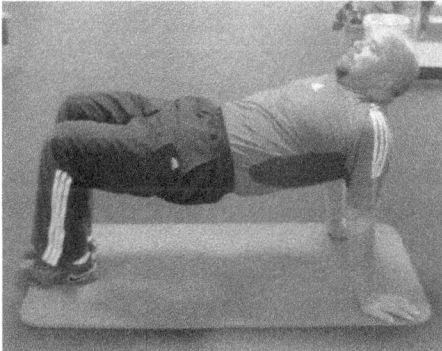

Chest

Exercise 2.1 – Pectoral Isometric hold

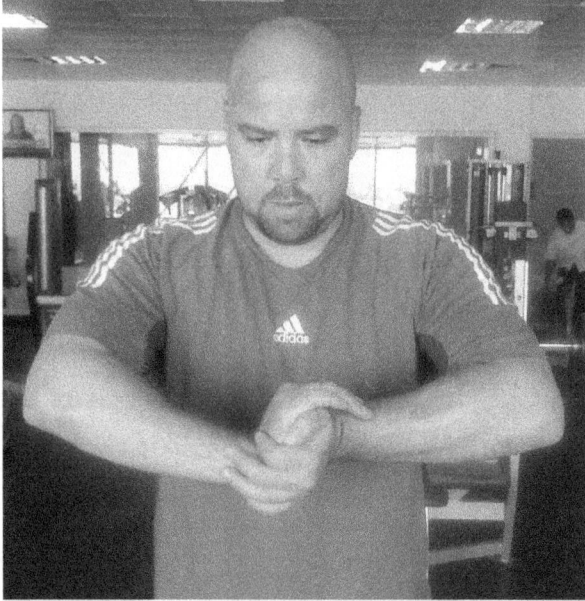

EXERCISE DESCRIPTION

Place your hands together & level with your chest and ensure that your shoulders are relaxed whilst pushing your hands towards each other. Breathe consistently whilst pushing harder and contract your abdominals accordingly to ensure that you increase the power for better results. Your hands should only be slightly in front of your body.

Exercise 2.2 – Incline Push Ups

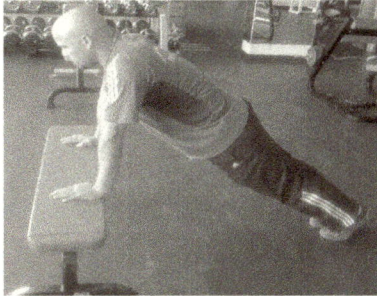

EXERCISE DESCRIPTION

Lean onto a bench/stable object ensuring that your back is straight and your hands are level with your shoulders. Your shoulders should be relaxed and your hips and shoulders should remain facing towards the ground along with your head and eyes. Initiate the movement from the abdominals and lower your upper body until your chest is close to the bench/stable object whilst breathing in. Breathe out as you raise your upper body back to the start position. Maintaining control throughout the movement is important whilst breathing correctly.

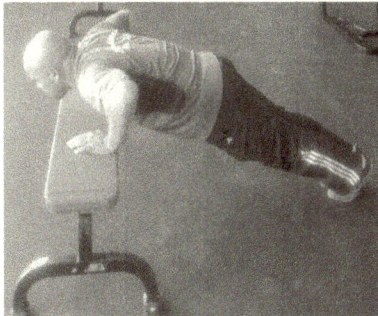

Exercise 2.3 – Normal Push Ups

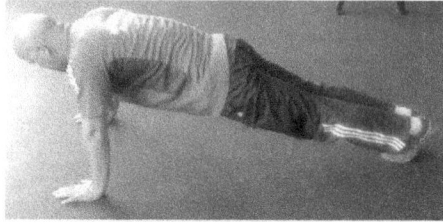

EXERCISE DESCRIPTION

From the kneeling position ensure that your hands are level with your shoulders and your knees and hands are in line. Your shoulders should be relaxed and your hips and shoulders should remain facing towards the ground along with your head and eyes. Initiate the movement from the abdominals and lower your upper body until your chest is close to the floor whilst breathing in. Breathe out as you raise your upper body back to the start position.

As you tire, concentrate on your breathing whilst compressing your abdominals and lower back; tense your whole body (not shoulders) to assist you in keeping good form. If this is too easy you can raise up from the floor whilst attempting to clap your hands together and return safely to the start position. Maintaining control throughout the movement is important whilst breathing correctly.

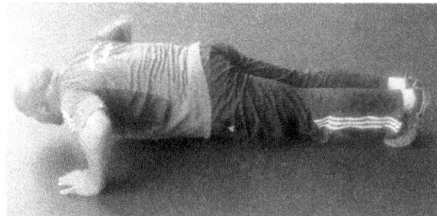

Exercise 2.4 – Decline Push Ups

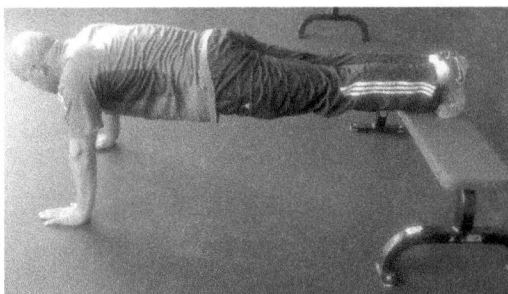

EXERCISE DESCRIPTION

With your feet on a stable raised object ensure your hands are level with your shoulders and your knees and hands are in line. Your shoulders should be relaxed and your hips and shoulders should remain facing towards the ground along with your head and eyes. Initiate the movement from the abdominals and lower your upper body until your chest is close to the floor whilst breathing in. Breathe out as you raise your upper body back to the start position. Maintaining control throughout the movement is important whilst breathing correctly.

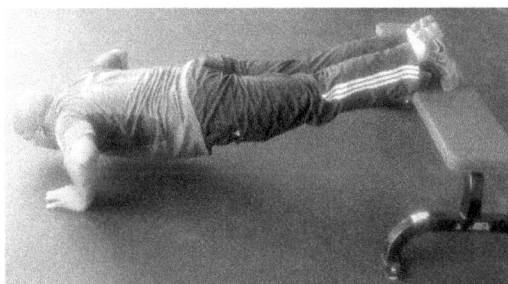

Exercise 2.5 – Bodyweight Dips

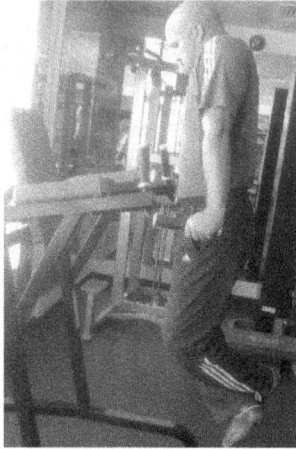

EXERCISE DESCRIPTION

Find any object that is stable, safe and secure where you can bend your elbows fully behind your body. Your aim is to place the chest in a fully stretched position before raising your body upwards whilst breathing out and straightening your arms. You can use the apparatus above or place a chair/raised platform behind you and complete the same exercise, although the above apparatus is better to get primary results for the chest as opposed to chest and triceps.

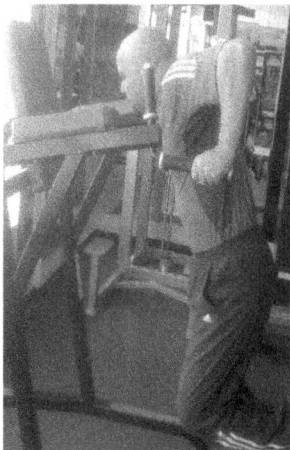

Shoulders

Exercise 3.1 – Isometric Holds 1-4

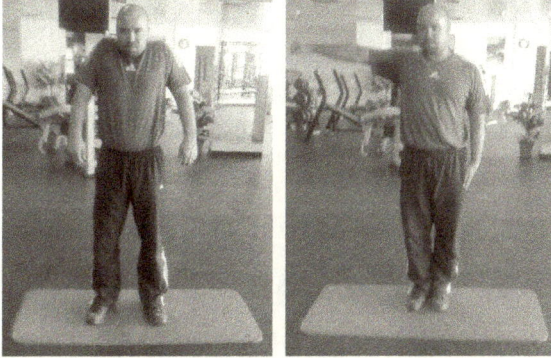

EXERCISE DESCRIPTION

Whichever hold you are doing you must ensure that wherever possible your posture is good i.e. maintaining body alignment with your head, eyes, shoulders and hips inline and facing forwards as much as possible. Your abdominals should be initiated prior and during each hold with your shoulders re-laxed as much as possible. All of the above movements are shoulder muscle actions; therefore all you are doing is moving the arm(s) in a particular direction and placing a hold within the range, your breathing should remain controlled and should not be forced.

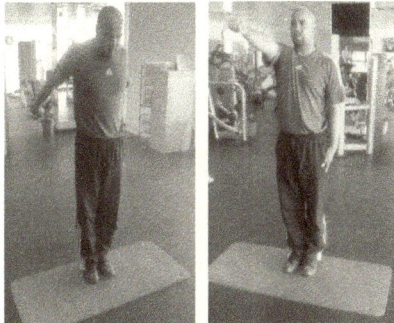

Exercise 3.2 – Advanced Hold

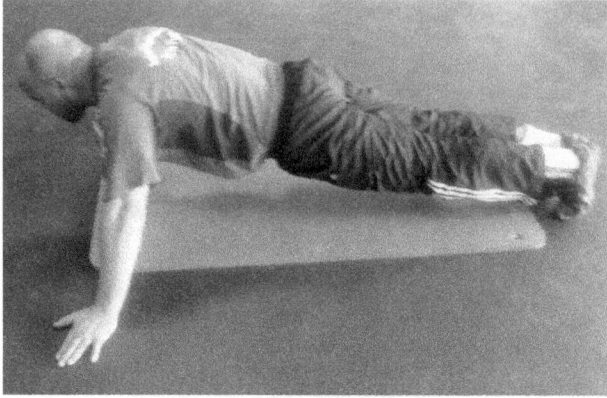

EXERCISE DESCRIPTION

With this hold you must ensure that your posture is perfect
i.e. maintaining body alignment with your head, eyes, shoulders and hips inline and facing forwards as much as possible.
Your abdominals should be initiated prior and during the hold
with your shoulders relaxed as much as possible. Your hands
should be inline with the shoulders and your breathing should
remain controlled and should not be forced. Hold the position
for as long as possible without disrupting your body alignment and good form.

Exercise 3.3 – Partner Resisted Exercises

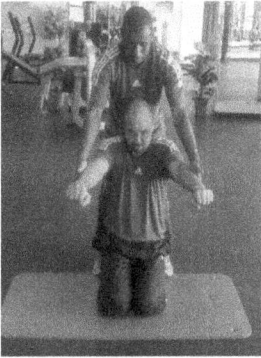 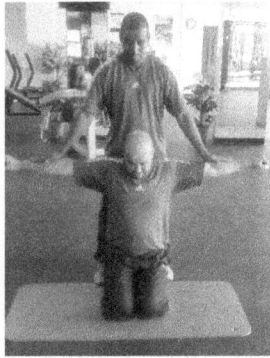

Pull arms down   Push arms up

EXERCISE DESCRIPTION

Most of the exercises shown are a variation of all the movements already covered (3.1), whether you are standing, or kneeling, your partner is just applying a resistance within a certain range whilst you attempt to raise, lower, push or pull against that resistance. You should always continue to breathe naturally and maintain good posture and form.

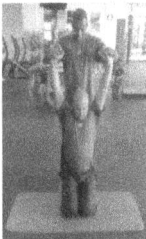 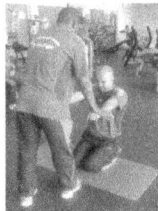 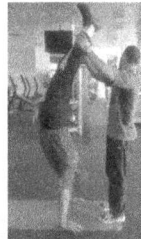

Push arms up   Push arms up   Hold or
                                Bend & Push

Exercise 3.4 – Caterpillar

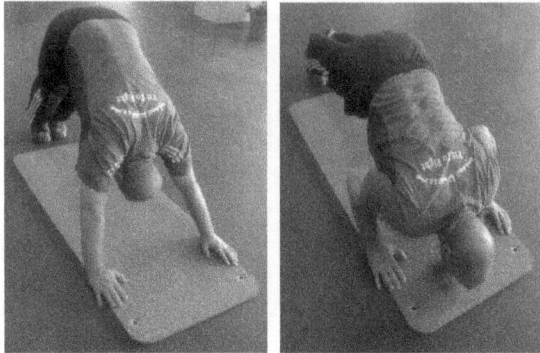

EXERCISE DESCRIPTION

With your toes on the floor, your hands level on the floor and around shoulder width apart, hold your body in a V position as best you can with your backside raised up slightly. Throughout all 3 movements your abdominals should be initiated and as you breathe out you should roll your bodyweight forwards using only your shoulders, roll down and forwards bending your arms at the elbows until your chest almost brushes the ground and then roll upwards straightening your arms and hold. Breathe in until you reverse the movement by rolling your shoulders in the opposite direction until you are back in the start position. Repeat the movement but keep the shoulders pulled down and backwards as much as possible which will ensure that your upper spine and head are relaxed and not under too much tension.

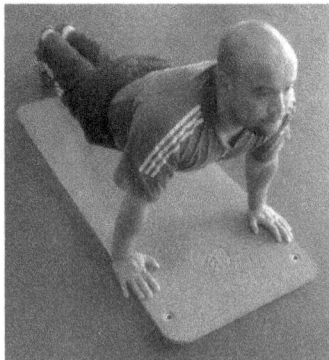

Exercise 3.5 – Additional Isometric Holds

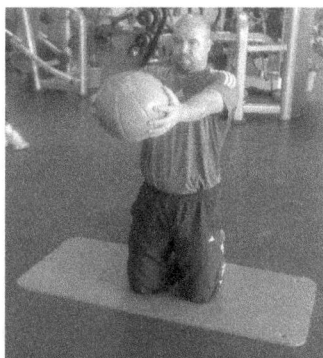

EXERCISE DESCRIPTION

Select a low enough resistance to start with until you have mastered the technique and position yourself in the kneeling or standing position. Whichever hold you are attempting your shoulders should be relaxed with your breathing as per normal. Initially you should breathe out, engage your abdominals and raise the weight up, out to the side or in front of you and hold for as long as you can throughout the different ranges of motion whilst maintaining good posture. When you feel your posture and good form faltering, control your breathing throughout but most importantly (in) as you return to the start position and repeat.

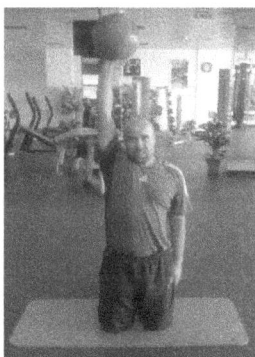

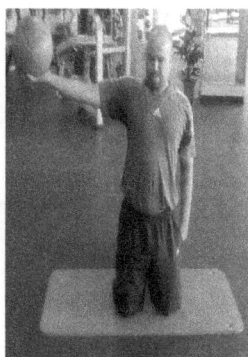

Biceps

Exercise 4.1 – Isometric hold

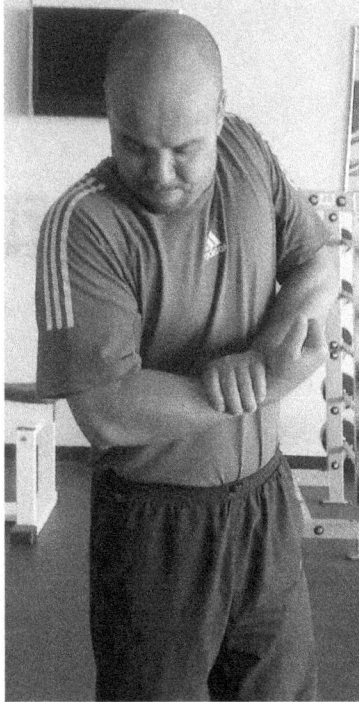

EXERCISE DESCRIPTION

Bend one of your elbows at any range and hold the wrist with your other hand, apply a resistance and attempt to fully bend your arm whilst applying a greater force. Try resisting throughout all of the ranges, hold and repeat.

Exercise 4.2 – Partner Resisted Holds

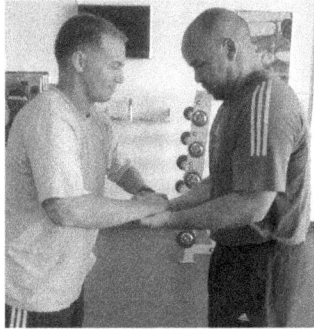

EXERCISE DESCRIPTION

Bend one or both of your elbows at any range whilst your partner holds your arm(s) ensure he/she applies a resistance as you attempt to fully bend your arm(s) as your partner applies a greater force. Try resisting throughout all of the ranges; hold and repeat (attempt both methods, left & right pictures).

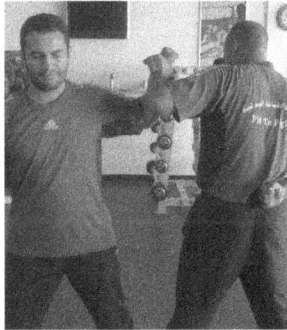

Exercise 4.3 – Under-grasp pull ups

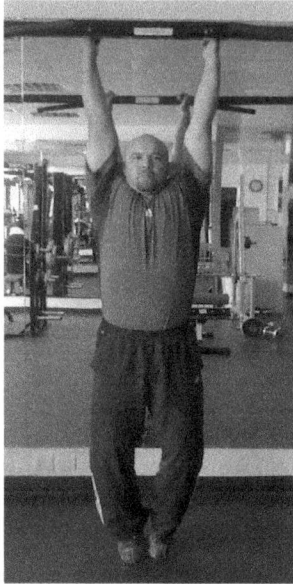

EXERCISE DESCRIPTION

Allow your body to hang in a straight line (under grasp) as you ensure that you have a tight grip on the pull up bar. Initiate your abdominals as you breathe out, pull your bodyweight up and attempt to get your chin above your hands whilst bending your arms only. Hold the position for 2-3 seconds, breathe in, lower your body under control and repeat.

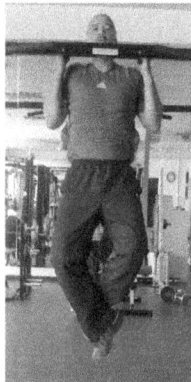

Exercise 4.4 – Behind the neck pull ups

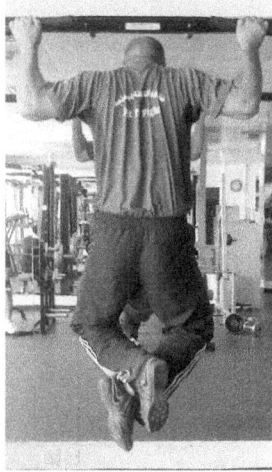

EXERCISE DESCRIPTION

Allow your body to hang in a straight line (wide grip) as you ensure that you have a tight grip on the pull up bar. Initiate your abdominals as you breathe out, pull your bodyweight up and attempt to get the back of your neck level with your hands whilst bending your arms only. Hold the position for 2-3 seconds, breathe in, lower your body under control and repeat.

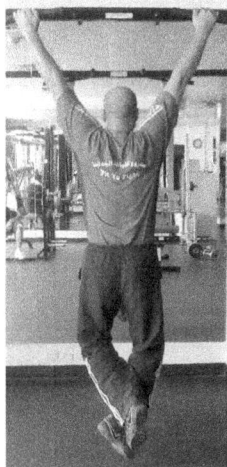

Triceps

Exercise 5.1 – Bench Dips

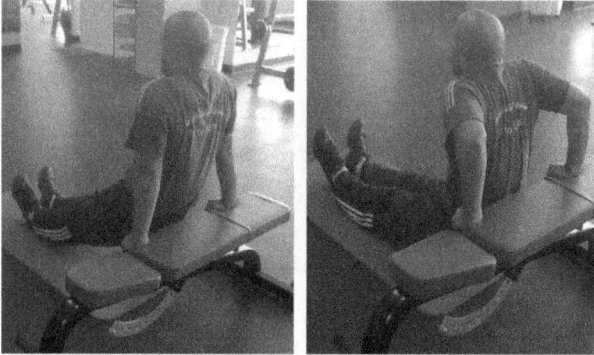

EXERCISE DESCRIPTION

Find any object that is stable, safe and secure where you can bend your elbows fully behind your body. Your aim is to place your hands firmly behind you on the bench and fairly close together. Start off with your arms straight before bending at the elbow as you breathe in, then as you breathe out raise your body upwards whilst contracting your triceps by straightening your arms. You can use the bench as above or place a chair/raised platform behind you and complete the same exercise, repeat the movement. Elevate your feet to make it more difficult.

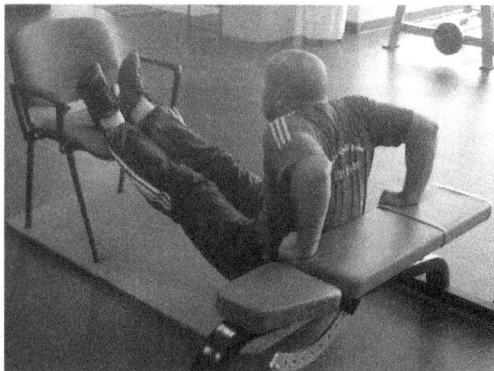

Exercise 5.2 – Incline press ups

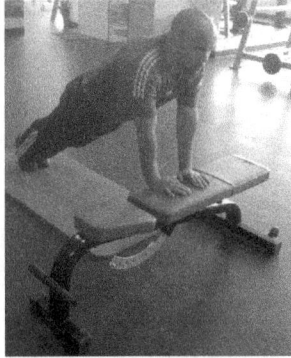

EXERCISE DESCRIPTION

Lean onto a bench/stable object ensuring that your back is straight and your shoulders relaxed whilst your hips and shoulders remain facing towards the ground along with your head and eyes. Place your hands close together before you initiate the movement from the abdominals and lower your upper body until your chest is close to the bench/stable object whilst breathing in. Breathe out as you raise your upper body back to the start position. Maintaining control throughout the movement is important whilst breathing correctly. It is very important to keep your elbows as close to the body as possible.

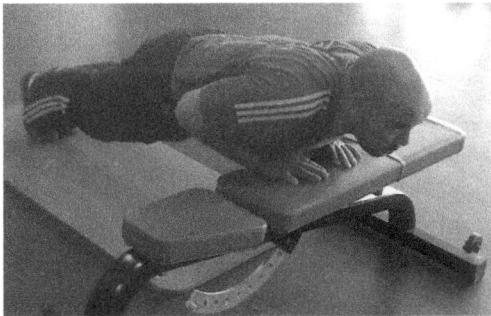

Exercise 5.3 – Advanced press ups

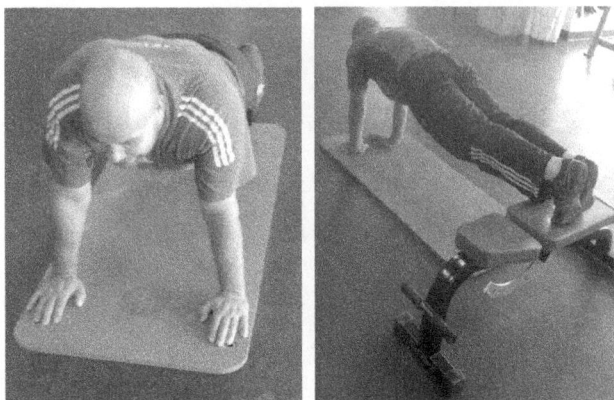

EXERCISE DESCRIPTION

With your feet on a stable raised object ensure your hands are initially level with your shoulders and your knees and hands are in line. Your shoulders should be relaxed and your hips and shoulders should remain facing towards the ground along with your head and eyes. Progress until your hands are as close together as possible before you initiate the movement from the abdominals and lower your upper body until your chest is close to the floor whilst breathing in. Breathe out as you raise your upper body back to the start position. Maintaining control throughout the movement is important whilst breathing correctly. It is very important to keep your elbows as close to the body as possible. Progress further by elevating the legs on a stable platform or unstable platform such as the fitball.

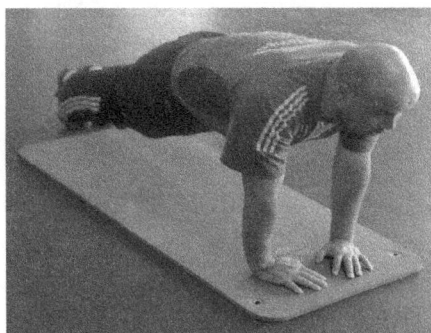

Exercise 5.4 – Partner walk

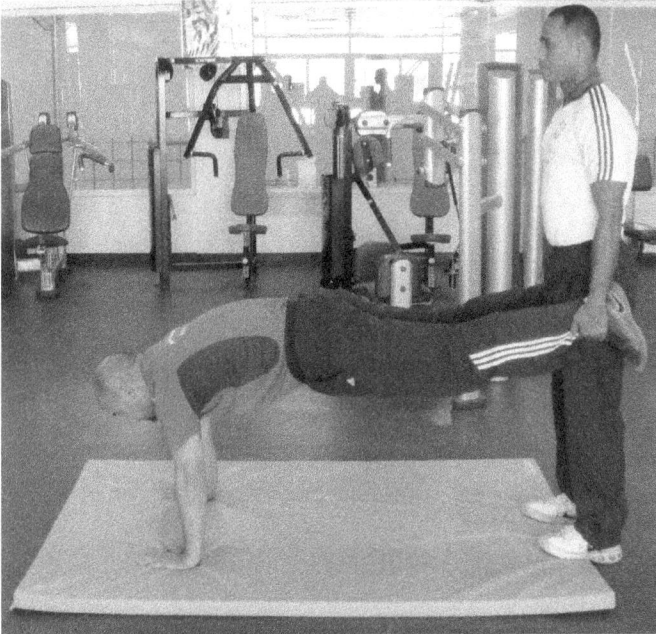

EXERCISE DESCRIPTION

Get in the press up position as your partner takes a good grip
of your legs, simply walk forwards in a straight line by using
your hands only. Before walking, initiate the abdominals and
endeavour to keep your back straight along with the head, eyes
hips and shoulders. Relax your shoulders as much as possible.

Exercise 5.5 – Body raises

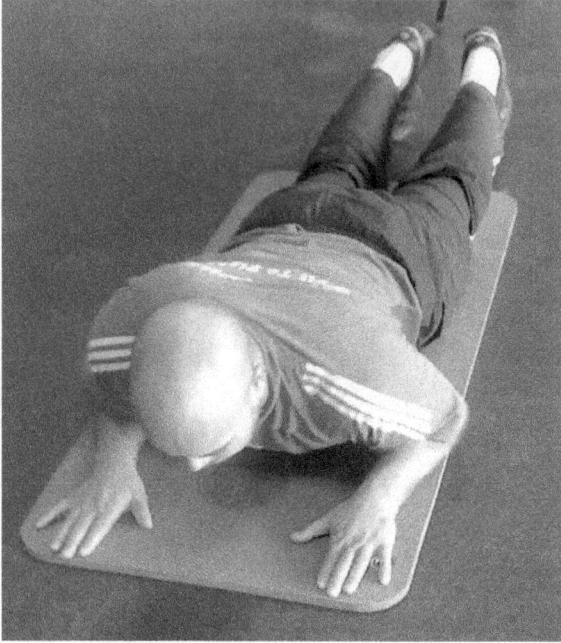

EXERCISE DESCRIPTION

Start in the front lying position with your hands level with your head shoulder width apart and with your elbows close to the sides of your body. Whilst using the arms only, initiate the abdominals and breathe out as you straighten your arms. Endeavour to keep your shoulders down and relaxed as much as possible.

Legs

Exercise 6.1 – Static Hold

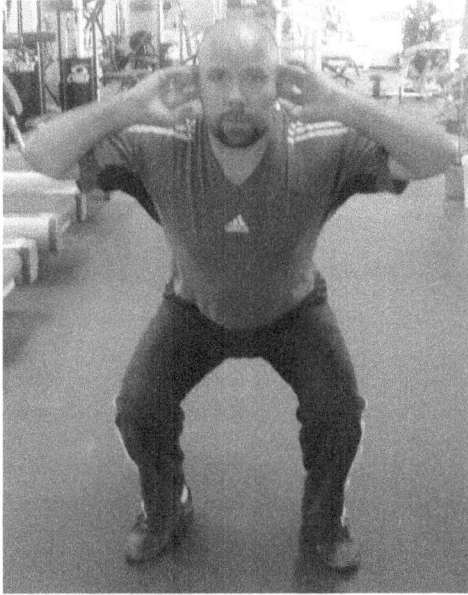

EXERCISE DESCRIPTION

Ensure that you stand with your feet flat on the floor and wide enough to maintain good balance, (normally shoulder width apart) your thighs should be parallel to the ground. Ensure your hips, shoulders, head and eyes are inline. Squat down and backwards until your knees are level with your toes. Hold the position for as long as you can, whilst breathing in a controlled manner.

Exercise 6.2 – Bridge

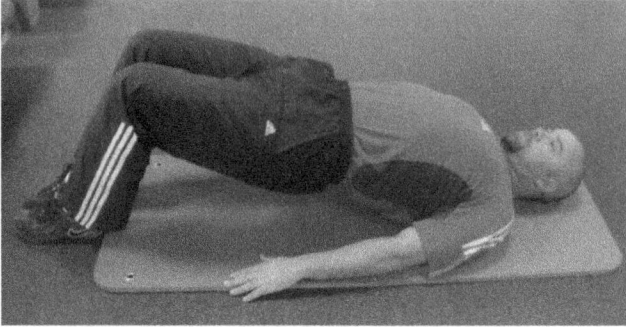

EXERCISE DESCRIPTION

In the back lying position place your feet shoulder width apart
and flat on the floor with your arms relaxed by your side. Your
hips, shoulders, head and eyes should be inline prior to raising
your hips off the ground whilst breathing out. Breathe in as
you return to the start position. Concentrate on maintaining a
good body position as you raise your hips high. Use the upper
leg muscles to hold you in the position. Repeat the movement
in a controlled manner.

Exercise 6.3 – Squat

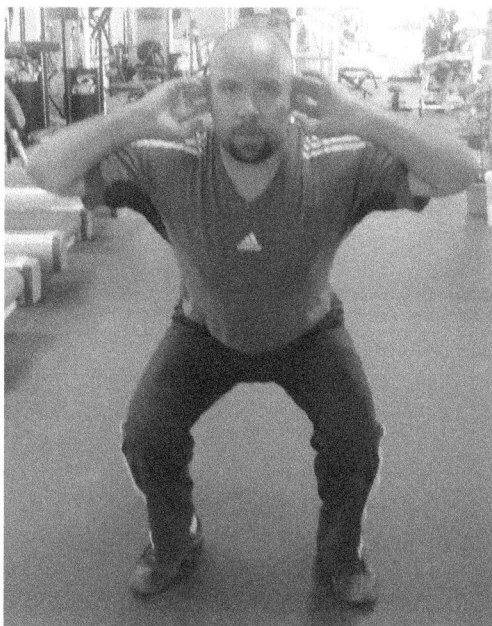

EXERCISE DESCRIPTION

Stand with your feet flat on the floor and wide enough to maintain good balance. Your hips, shoulders, head and eyes should be inline as you squat down keeping your back straight, squat down and backwards until your thighs are parallel to the ground. Ensure your knees don't go too far beyond your toes as you hold the position for 2-3 seconds before returning to the start position. Breathe in a controlled manner.

Exercise 6.4 – Lunge

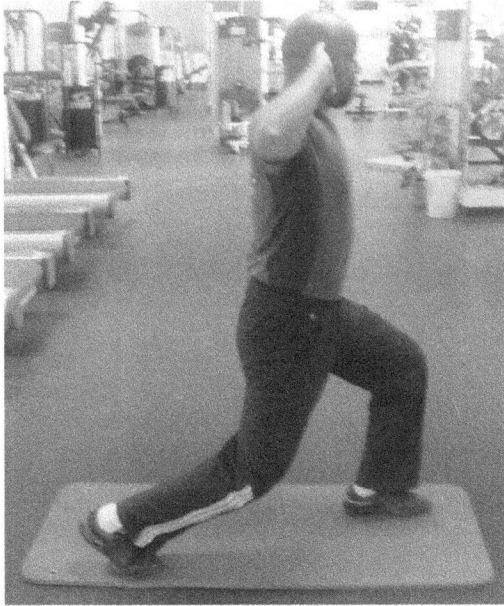

EXERCISE DESCRIPTION

Stand with your feet flat on the floor and wide enough to
maintain good balance. Step backwards with one leg until the
thigh of the forward leg is parallel to the ground, your hips,
shoulders, head and eyes should be inline and facing forwards.
Initiate the movement via the abdominals whilst keeping the
back straight and breathing out, breathe in as you return to the
start position and repeat. All movements should be under control and safe!! This exercise can be changed so that you step
forwards instead.

Exercise 6.5 – Step Up

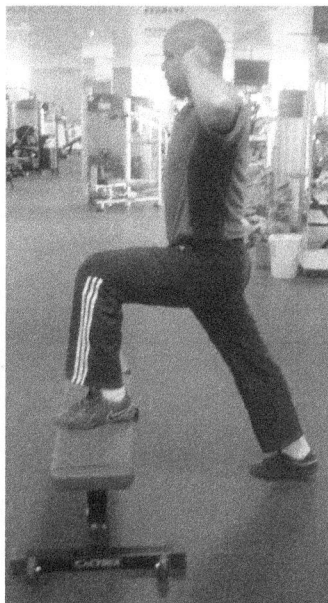

EXERCISE DESCRIPTION

Stand with your feet flat on the floor and wide enough to maintain good balance. Choose a surface that is not too low or too high and your foot is flat on it before you step up. Your hips, shoulders, head and eyes should be inline and facing forwards. Initiate the movement via the abdominals and breathe out when you step up and attempt to stand upright. As always it is very important that your back remains straight at all times. Breathe in as you return to the start position and repeat. All movements should be under control and safe!!

Exercise 6.6 – Squat Jump

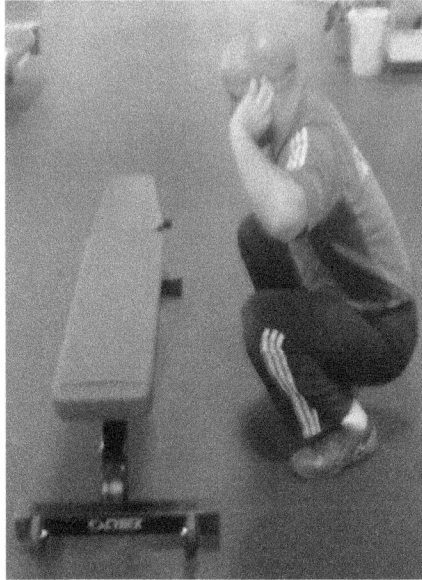

EXERCISE DESCRIPTION

Choose a stable surface to use for this exercise and start off with it up against a wall. Stand with your feet flat on the floor and wide enough to maintain good balance. Your hips, shoulders, head and eyes should be inline as you squat down keeping your back straight, squat down and backwards until your thighs are close to the ground. Breathe out as you jump forward and upwards onto the stable surface. Progress in a safe manner onto a low surface first and gradually increase the height as you become more confident. Initiating the abdominals, keeping the back straight and your breathing are very important factors whilst attempting this exercise.

Full bodyweight program – (template)

Back exercises	Reps	Sets	Remarks
Back extensions			
Alt arm/leg raise 1&2			
Straight leg hold			
Plank progressions			
Hip raises			
Chest exercises	**Reps**	**Sets**	**Remarks**
Isometric hold			
Incline Push Ups			
Normal Push Ups			
Decline Push Ups			
Bodyweight Dips			
Shoulder exercises	**Reps**	**Sets**	**Remarks**
Isometric holds 1-4			
Advanced Hold			
Partner Resisted Ex's			
Caterpillar			
Additional Holds			
Bicep exercises	**Reps**	**Sets**	**Remarks**
Isometric hold			
Partner Res Holds			
Under-grasp pull ups			
Behind neck pull ups			
Triceps exercises	**Reps**	**Sets**	**Remarks**
Bench Dips			
Incline Press Ups			
Advanced press ups			
Partner walk			
Body raises			
Leg exercises	**Reps**	**Sets**	**Remarks**
Static Hold			
Bridge			
Squat			
Lunge			
Step Up			
Squat Jump			

RESISTANCE BAND EX'S

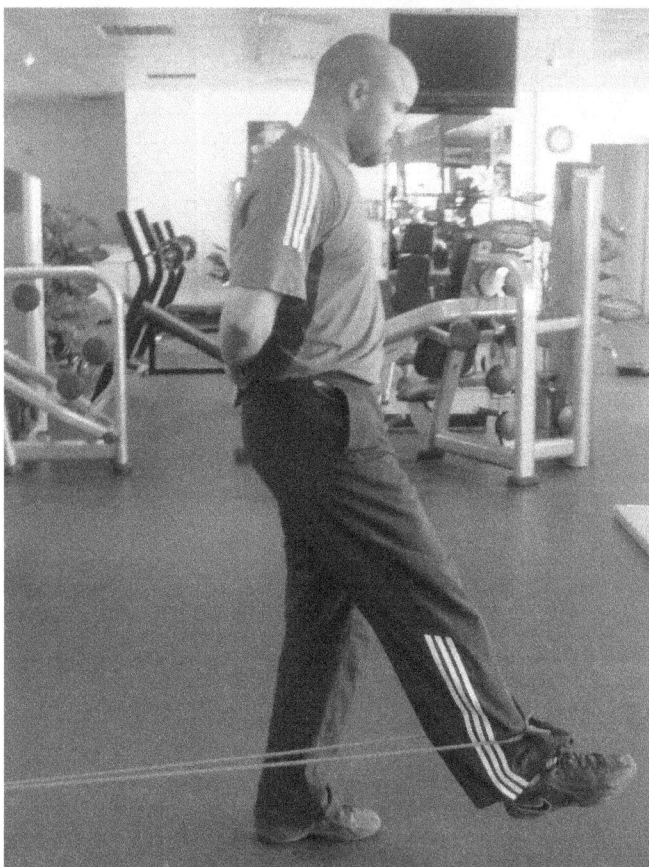

Chapter 4

Back

Exercise 1.1 – Single arm row

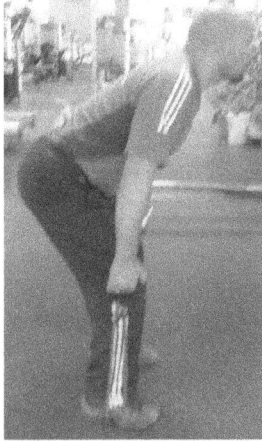

EXERCISE DESCRIPTION

Firstly, choose a band that is the correct resistance for you and during the initial stages this will be a light weight until you master the technique. Stand with your feet flat on the floor and around shoulder width apart, stand on the band until there is enough tension for your back muscles to resist. Your hips, shoulders, head and eyes should be in line with a slight bend at the waist and knees. Start off with your arm straight whilst holding onto the band and pull it towards your waist whilst breathing out ensuring your elbow is close to the side of your body. Attempt to initiate the movement via your abdominals but use your back muscles to pull the band up with as little assistance from the biceps as possible. Return to the start position whilst breathing in and repeat accordingly.

Exercise 1.2 – Bent over row

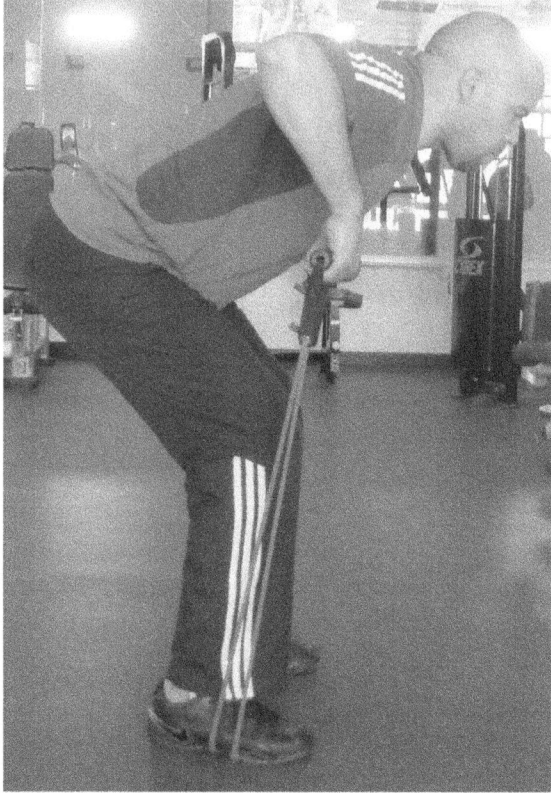

EXERCISE DESCRIPTION

Firstly, choose a band that is the correct resistance for you and during the initial stages this will be a light weight until you master the technique. Stand with your feet flat on the floor and around shoulder width apart, stand on the band until there is enough tension for your back muscles to resist. Your hips, shoulders, head and eyes should be inline, with a slight bend at the waist and knees. Start off with your arms straight whilst holding onto the band and pull it towards your waist whilst breathing out ensuring your elbows are close to the side of your body. Attempt to initiate the movement via your abdominals but use your back muscles to pull the band up with as little assistance from the biceps as possible. Return to the start position whilst breathing in and repeat accordingly.

Exercise 1.3 – Seated row

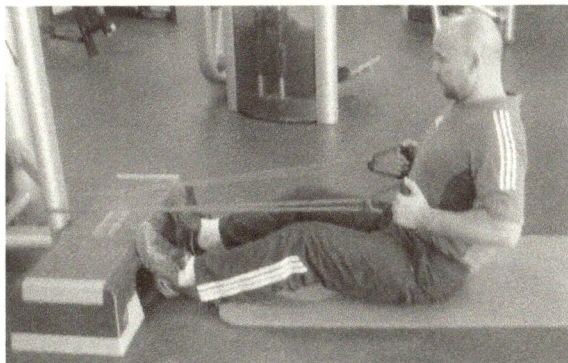

EXERCISE DESCRIPTION

Firstly, choose a band that is the correct resistance for you and during the initial stages this will be a light weight until you master the technique. The band should be securely fitted around a solid object around waist height (whilst sitting). Sit with your legs outstretched on the floor and up against an object to ensure that there is a slight bend at your knees. The band should have enough tension for your back muscles to resist. Your hips, shoulders, head and eyes should be inline and you should start off leaning slightly forwards with your arms straight whilst holding onto the band and pull it towards your waist whilst breathing out ensuring your elbows are close to the side of your body. Attempt to initiate the movement via your abdominals but use your back muscles to pull the band towards you with as little assistance from the biceps as possible. Return to the start position whilst breathing in and repeat accordingly.

Exercise 1.4 – Lat pull down

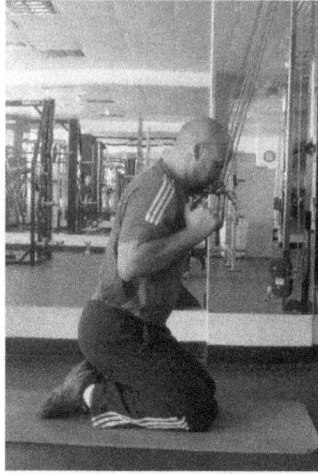

EXERCISE DESCRIPTION

Firstly, choose a band that is the correct resistance for you and during the initial stages this will be a light weight until you master the technique. The band should be securely fitted around a solid object above head height. Kneel down on the floor and make sure the band has enough tension for your back muscles to resist. Your hips, shoulders, head and eyes should be inline and you should start off with the band above and in front of you. Your arms should start off straight whilst holding onto the band and then pull it towards your waist whilst breathing out ensuring your elbows are close to the side of your body. Attempt to initiate the movement via your abdominals but use your back muscles to pull the band towards you with as little assistance from the biceps as possible. Return to the start position whilst breathing in and repeat accordingly.

Exercise 1.5 – Reverse flyes

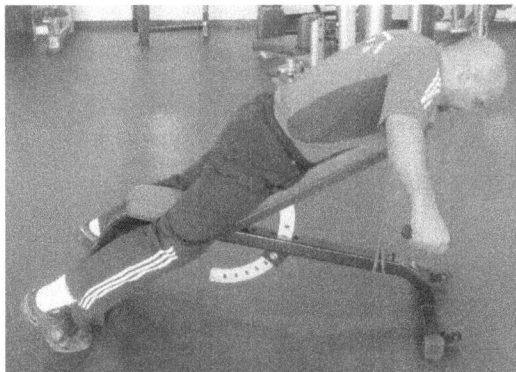

EXERCISE DESCRIPTION

Firstly, choose a band that is the correct resistance for you and during the initial stages this will be a light weight until you master the technique. The band should be securely fitted around a solid object below you around chest height. Lean onto an inclined bench and make sure the band has enough tension for your back muscles to resist. Your hips, shoulders, head and eyes should be inline, and you should start off with your arms almost straight and towards the ground. Pull the band towards you whilst breathing out ensuring your elbows are slightly bent. Attempt to initiate the movement via your abdominals but use your upper back muscles to pull the band towards you as if you are bringing your shoulder blades together. There should be as little assistance from the shoulders as possible (no tension). Return to the start position whilst breathing in and repeat accordingly. This exercise can also be done on a bench that has less of an incline or in the standing position.

Chest

Exercise 2.1 – Chest Press

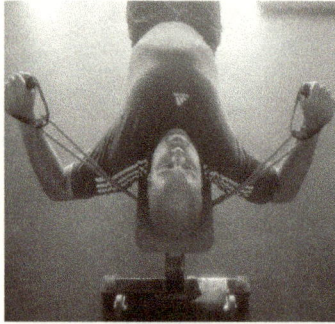

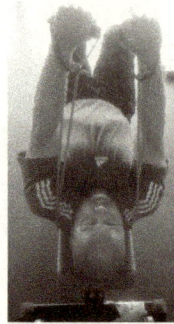

EXERCISE DESCRIPTION

Safety should be your main priority especially when selecting the weight of the resistance band until you have mastered the technique and ensure that you secure the band safely around a solid object. Position yourself either on a flat surface or in the kneeling position and grip the bands firmly with one or both hands depending on the exercise. Once you have adjusted the resistance so that it is taught enough, position your hands level with the upper part of your chest with your elbows low where possible. As you breathe out, engage your abdominals and push the bands away from your body whilst straightening your arm(s). Breathe in as you return to the start position and repeat.

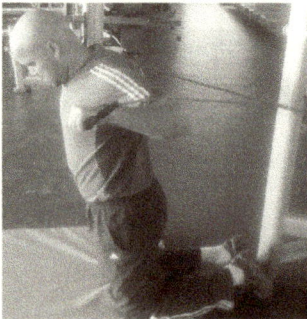

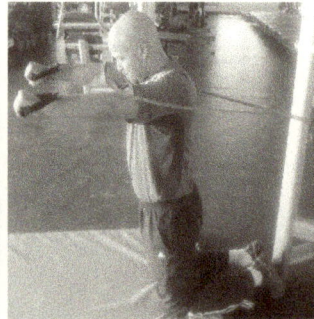

Exercise 2.2 – Flyes 1

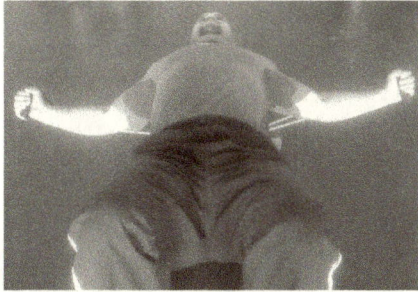

EXERCISE DESCRIPTION

Safety should be your main priority especially when selecting the weight of the resistance band until you have mastered the technique and ensure that you secure the band safely around a solid object. Position yourself on a flat surface and grip the bands firmly with one or both hands depending on the exercise. Once you have adjusted the resistance so that it is taught enough, position your hands level with the upper part of your chest with your elbows low where possible and positioned out to the side of your body with outstretched arm(s) slightly below the level of your shoulder. As you breathe out, engage your abdominals and pull the bands up towards the midline of your body. Breathe in as you return to the start position and repeat. Attempt to keep your arm(s) straight albeit with a very slight bend at the elbow.

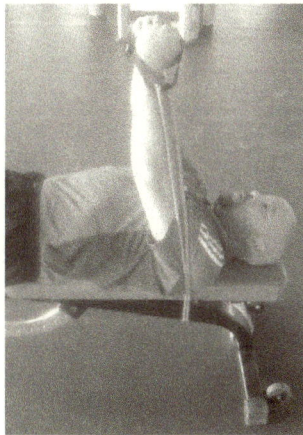

Exercise 2.3 – Flyes 2 & 3

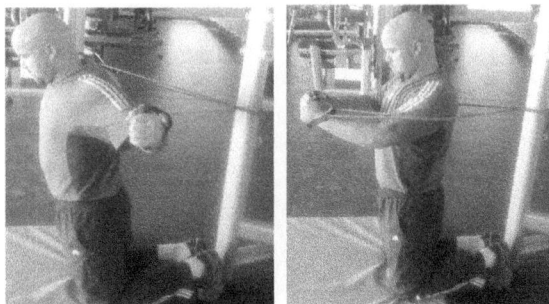

EXERCISE DESCRIPTION

Safety should be your main priority especially when selecting the weight of the resistance band until you have mastered the technique and ensure that you secure the band safely around a solid object. Position yourself on your knees and grip the bands firmly with one or both hands depending on the exercise. Once you have adjusted the resistance so that it is taught enough, position your hands level with the upper part of your chest with your elbows low where possible and positioned out to the side of your body with outstretched arm(s) slightly below the level of your shoulder. As you breathe out, engage your abdominals and pull the bands forwards towards the midline of your body.

Breathe in as you return to the start position and repeat. Attempt to keep a very slight bend at the elbow. Lean forward to work your chest at a different angle.

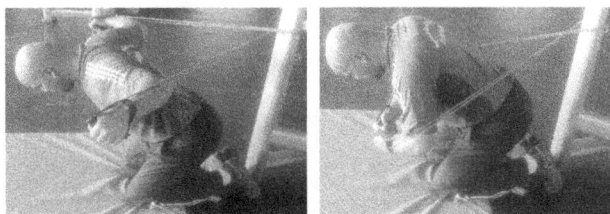

Exercise 2.4 – Pullovers

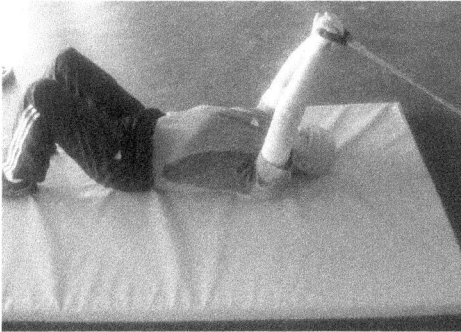

EXERCISE DESCRIPTION

Select a safe weight to start with until you have mastered the technique and position yourself on a flat surface, preferably a mat or a bench and grip the band firmly with one or both hands depending on the exercise. Your arm(s) should be above your head and as you breathe out, engage your abdominals and pull the bands towards your hips. Your arm(s) should remain as straight as is comfortable, breathe in as you return to the start position and repeat.

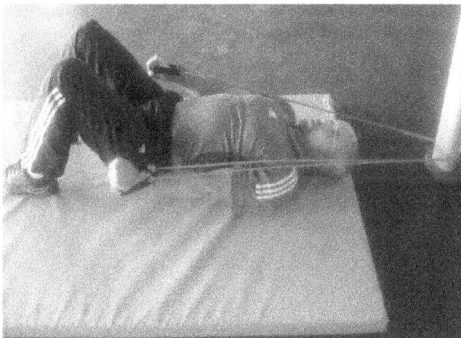

Shoulders

Exercise 3.1 – Isometric Holds

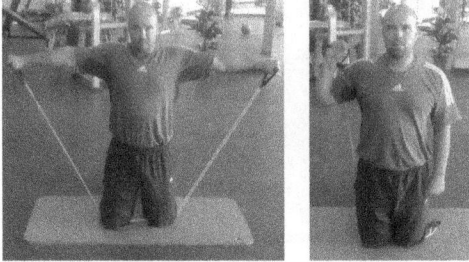

EXERCISE DESCRIPTION

Select a low enough resistance to start with until you have mastered the technique and position yourself in the kneeling or standing position with the band secure & evenly fixed. Grip the band(s) firmly with one or both hands. Whichever hold you are attempting your shoulders should be relaxed with your breathing as per normal. Initially you should breathe out, engage your abdominals and raise the bands up, out to the side or behind you and hold for as long as you can throughout the different ranges of motion whilst maintaining good posture. When you feel your posture and good form faltering, control your breathing throughout but most importantly (in) as you return to the start position and repeat.

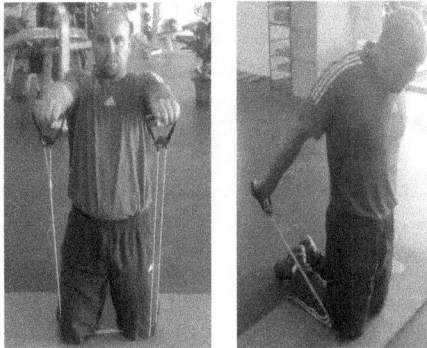

Exercise 3.2 – Shoulder Press

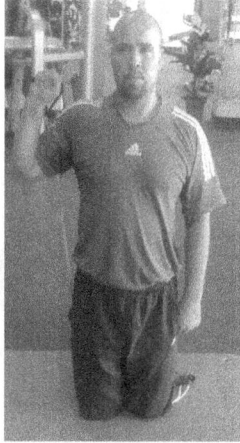

EXERCISE DESCRIPTION

Select a low enough resistance to start with until you have
mastered the technique and position yourself in the kneeling or
standing position with the band secure & evenly fixed. Grip
the band(s) firmly with one or both hands. Initially the bands
should be positioned on either the front or rear of your shoulders with your elbows low and close to the side of your body.
As you breathe out, engage your abdominals and raise the
bands up and above your head with your arms outstretched
and hold. Attempt to keep the bands level, along with keeping
your arm(s) straight, breathe in as you return to the start position and repeat.

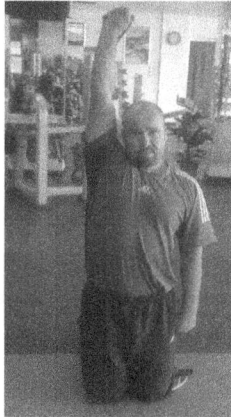

Exercise 3.3 – Frontal Raise

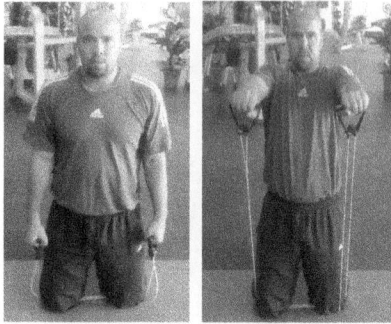

EXERCISE DESCRIPTION

Select a low enough resistance to start with until you have mastered the technique and position yourself in the kneeling or standing position with the band secure & evenly fixed. Grip the band(s) firmly with one or both hands. Initially the bands should be positioned down and close to the front of the body with one or both arm(s) straight. As you breathe out, engage your abdominals and raise the bands up and level with your shoulders and hold. Attempt to keep the bands level along with keeping your arm(s) straight albeit with a very slight bend at the elbow to avoid injury. Breathe in as you return to the start position and repeat.

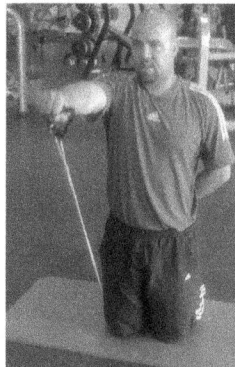

Exercise 3.4 – Rear Deltoid

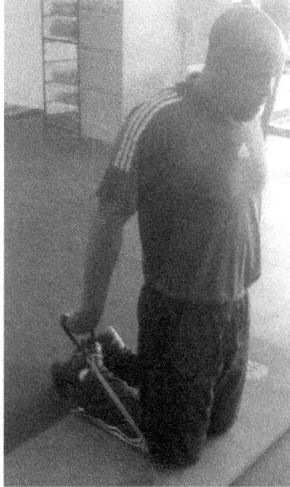

EXERCISE DESCRIPTION

Select a low enough resistance to start with until you have
mastered the technique and position yourself in the kneeling or
standing position with the band secure & evenly fixed. Grip
the band(s) firmly with one or both hands. As you breathe out,
engage your abdominals and raise the bands away from the
rear of your body and hold. Attempt to keep the band(s) level
along with keeping your arms straight attempt to relax the
shoulders and stick your chest out, breathe in as you return to
the start position and repeat.

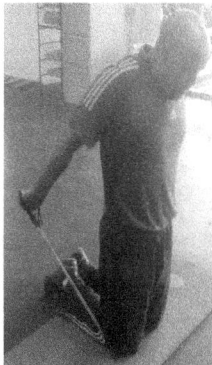

Exercise 3.5 – Lateral Raise

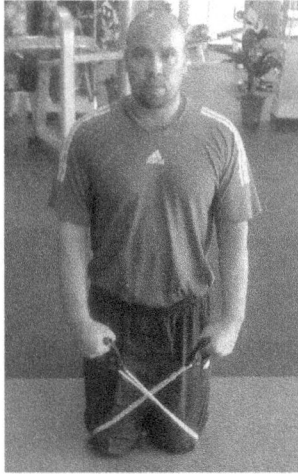

EXERCISE DESCRIPTION

Select a low resistance to start with until you have mastered
the technique and position yourself in the kneeling or standing
position with the band secure, twisted but evenly fixed. Grip
the bands firmly with both hands and the bands positioned
down and close to the side of your body with straight arms. As
you breathe out, engage your abdominals and raise the bands
up, level with your shoulders with outstretched arms and hold.
Attempt to keep the bands level and your arms straight albeit
with a very slight bend at the elbow to avoid injury. Breathe in
as you return to the start position and repeat.

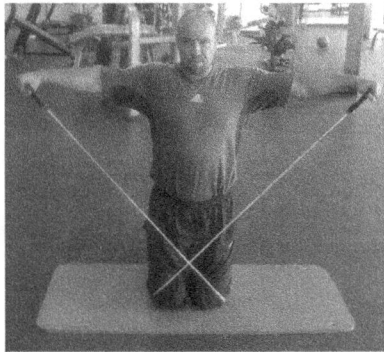

Biceps

Exercise 4.1 – Isometric Hold

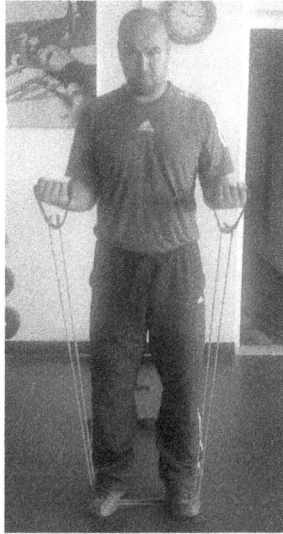

EXERCISE DESCRIPTION

Select a safe resistance to start with until you have mastered
the technique and position yourself in the standing upright
position with your legs around shoulder width apart, slightly
bent and level. Grip the resistance bands firmly with both
hands and close to the side of your body with straight arms. As
you breathe out, engage your abdominals and raise the bands
up to the midway position by bending your elbows and hold.
Attempt to hold for a long enough period and then breathe in
as you slowly return to the start position and repeat.

Exercise 4.2 – Standing Curls

Both arms

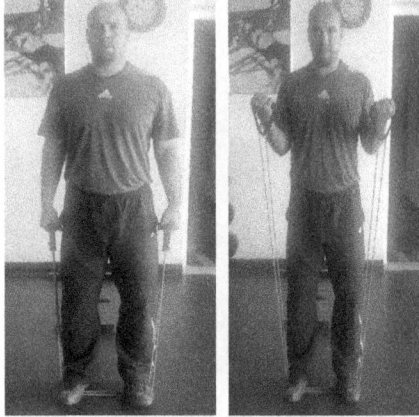

EXERCISE DESCRIPTION

Select a safe resistance to start with until you have mastered the technique and position yourself in the standing upright position with your legs around shoulder width apart, slightly bent and level. Grip the resistance bands firmly with both hands and positioned down and close to the side of your body with straight arms. As you breathe out, engage your abdominals and raise the bands up fully by bending your elbows and hold. Attempt to keep the bands level and breathe in as you slowly return to the start position and repeat.

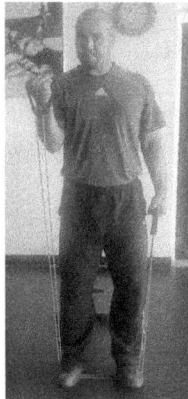

Single arm

94

Exercise 4.3 – Overhead Pull

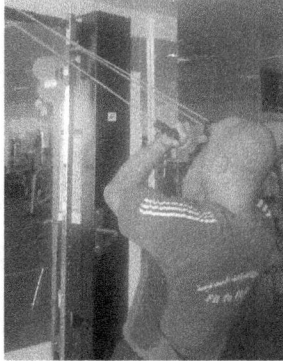

EXERCISE DESCRIPTION

Select a safe resistance to start with until you have mastered the technique and position yourself in the standing position (leaning back slightly) with your legs around shoulder width apart, slightly bent and level. Hook the bands overhead to a sturdy object and grip the resistance bands firmly with both hands. Position the bands in front of you and above your head with straight arms (picture below). As you breathe out, engage your abdominals and pull the bands towards you fully by bending your elbows and hold. Attempt to keep the bands level and breathe in as you slowly return to the start position and repeat.

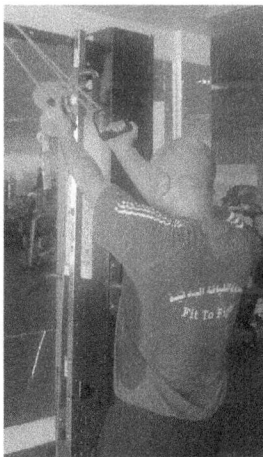

Exercise 4.4 – Bent over curl

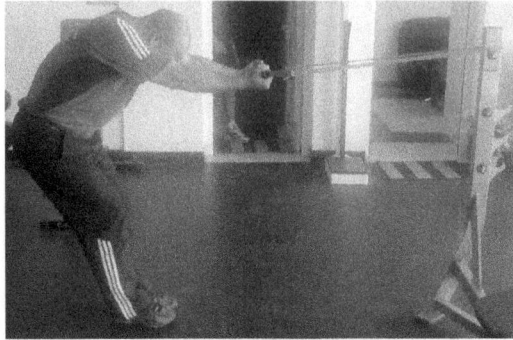

EXERCISE DESCRIPTION

Select a safe resistance to start with until you have mastered the technique and position yourself in the standing position (bent over slightly) with your legs in a balanced stance, slightly bent and level. Hook the bands to a sturdy object around chest height and grip the resistance bands firmly with both hands. Position the bands in front of you and ensure your arms are straight (picture above). As you breathe out, engage your abdominals and pull the bands towards you fully by bending your elbows and hold. Attempt to keep the bands level and breathe in as you slowly return to the start position and repeat.

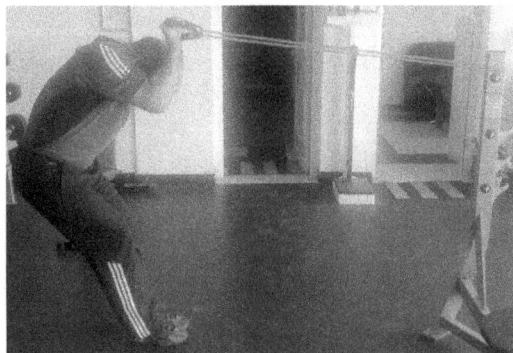

Triceps

Exercise 5.1 – Kneeling overhead press

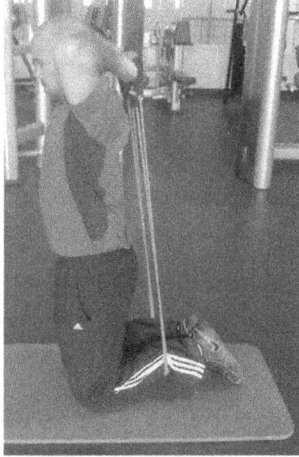

EXERCISE DESCRIPTION

Select a safe resistance to start with until you have mastered the technique and position yourself in the kneeling or standing position. Ensure that the band is secure and has enough tension before you begin. Start with your arms fully bent at the elbows behind your head, initiate the abdominals as you breathe out and raise the bands above your head contracting your triceps as you straighten the arms. Breathe in & return back to the start position under control, repeat the movement.

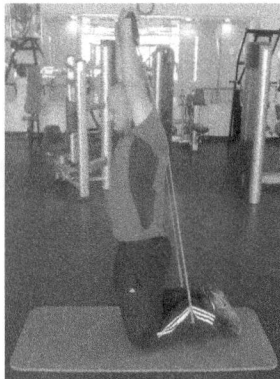

Exercise 5.2 – Kickbacks

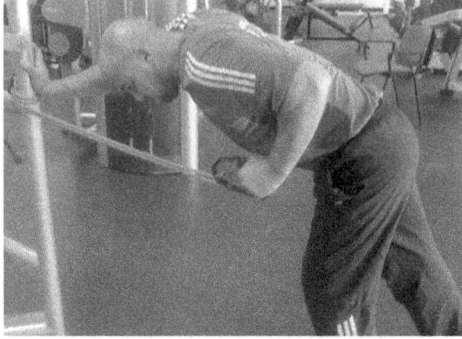

EXERCISE DESCRIPTION

Select a safe resistance to start with until you have mastered the technique and position yourself in the standing position, leaning slightly forwards. Ensure that the band is secure and has enough tension before you begin. Start with one arm resting (for stability) and the other arm bent at the elbow with the band close to the body. Breathe out as you straighten the arm behind you whilst contracting your triceps, breathe in as you return the band back to the start position and change arms as you repeat the movement.

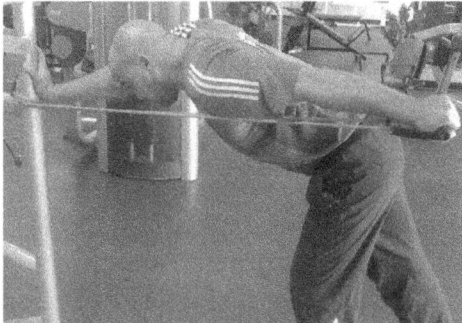

Exercise 5.3 – Over-head push

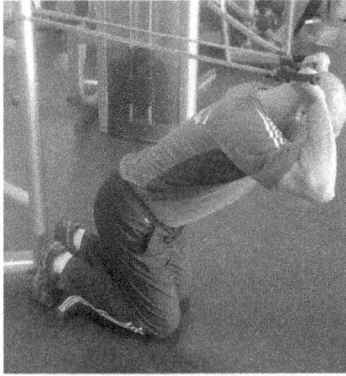

EXERCISE DESCRIPTION

Select a safe resistance to start with until you have mastered the technique and position yourself in the kneeling position. Ensure that the band is secure and has enough tension before you begin. Start with your arms fully bent at the elbows behind your head, initiate the abdominals as you breathe out and push the bands in front of your head contracting your triceps as you straighten the arms. Breathe in & return back to the start position under control, repeat the movement. Move the arms only and relax the shoulders.

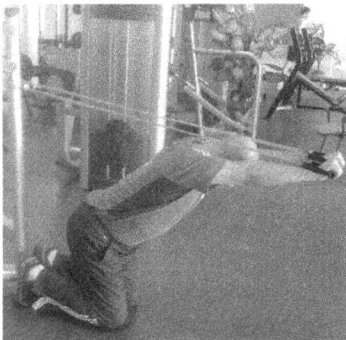

Exercise 5.4 – Forward press

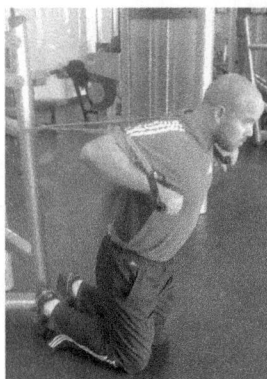

EXERCISE DESCRIPTION

Select a safe resistance to start with until you have mastered the technique and position yourself in the kneeling position. Ensure that the band is secure and has enough tension before you begin. Start with your elbows behind you, shoulder blades close together with your hands holding the handles close to your chest. Initiate the abdominals as you breathe out and push the bands forwards as you straighten your arms to contract your triceps. Breathe in as you return back to the start position and repeat the movement.

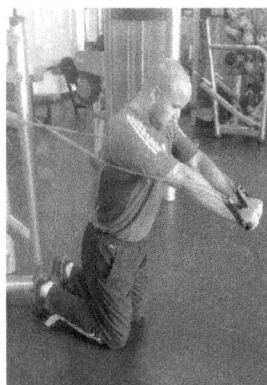

Legs

Exercise 6.1 – Squats

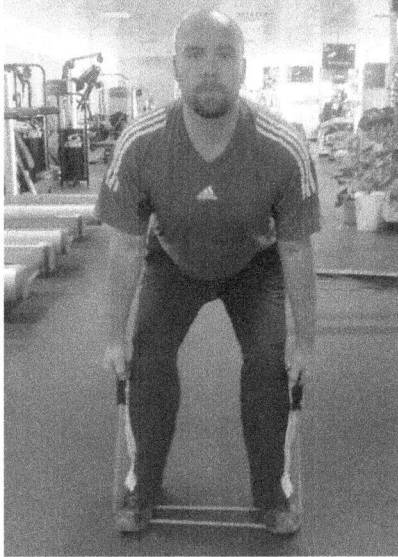

EXERCISE DESCRIPTION

Firstly, choose a band that is the correct resistance for you and during the initial stages this will be a light weight until you master the technique. Stand with your feet flat on the floor and wide enough to maintain good balance with the band secure & under your feet. Your hips, shoulders, head and eyes should be inline as you squat down keeping your back straight, squat down and backwards until your thighs are parallel to the ground. Ensure your knees don't go too far beyond your toes as you hold the position for 2-3 seconds before returning to the start position. Breathe in a controlled manner.

Exercise 6.2 – Hip extension

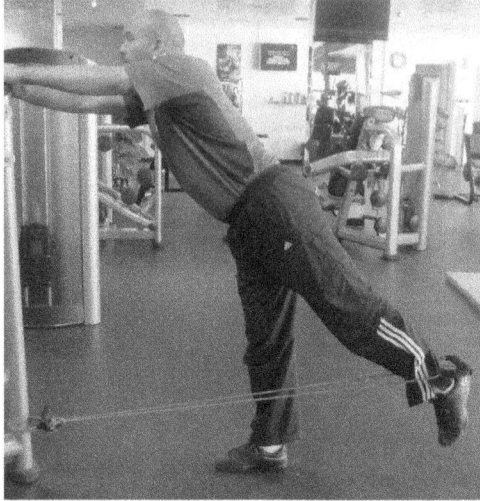

EXERCISE DESCRIPTION

Firstly, choose a band that is the correct resistance for you and during the initial stages this will be a light weight until you master the technique. Attach the band to one of your legs whilst ensuring your other foot is firmly stable on the ground. Begin by holding onto something as you progress the exercise, although your aim should be to not do so and this will also work the stationary leg. Begin by standing as upright as possible, initiate your abdominals and pull the cable away from the midline of the body whilst breathing out. Breathe in as you return to the start position under control and repeat accordingly. Your leg should be as straight as possible. As you progress you can place your arms out to the side, by your side or across your chest.

Exercise 6.3 – Hip flexion

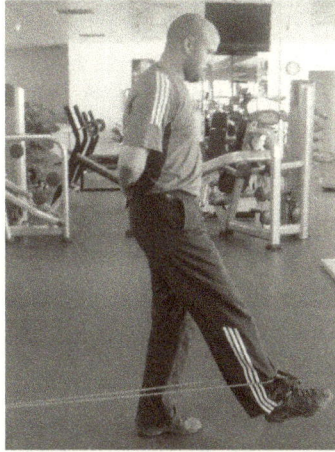

EXERCISE DESCRIPTION

Firstly, choose a band that is the correct resistance for you and during the initial stages this will be a light weight until you master the technique. Attach the band to one of your legs whilst ensuring your other foot is firmly stable on the ground. Begin by holding onto something as you progress the exercise, although your aim should be to not do so and this will also work the stationary leg. Begin by standing as upright as possible, initiate your abdominals and pull the cable away from the midline of the body whilst breathing out. Breathe in as you return to the start position under control and repeat accordingly. Your leg should be as straight as possible. As you progress you can place your arms out to the side, by your side or across your chest.

103

Exercise 6.4 – Abduction / Adduction

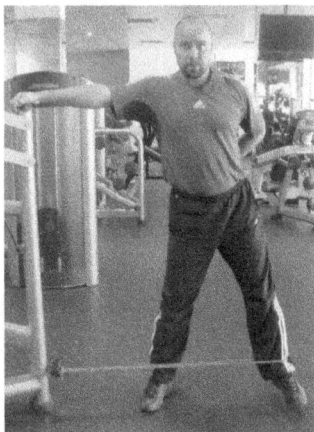

EXERCISE DESCRIPTION

Firstly, choose a band that is the correct resistance for you and during the initial stages this will be a light weight until you master the technique. Attach the band to one of your legs whilst ensuring your other foot is firmly stable on the ground. Begin by holding onto something as you progress the exercise, although your aim should be to not do so and this will also work the stationary leg. Begin by standing as upright as possible, initiate your abdominals and pull the cable away from the midline of the body whilst breathing out. Breathe in as you return to the start position under control and repeat accordingly. Your leg should be as straight as possible. As you progress you can place your arms out to the side, by your side or across your chest.

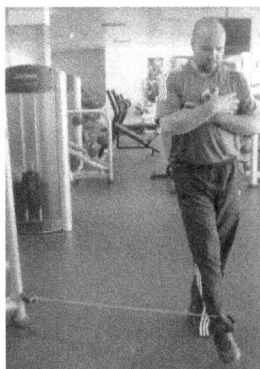

Resistance band program template

Each band has a different strength and colour e.g. Yellow = light, green = Medium and red = heavy. You must ensure that the band is secure before commencing each exercise.

Colour band used (_____)

Back exercises	Reps	Sets	Remarks
Single arm row			
Bent over row			
Seated row			
Lat pull down			
Reverse flyes			
Chest exercises	**Reps**	**Sets**	**Remarks**
Chest Press			
Flyes 1			
Flyes 2 & 3			
Pullovers			
Shoulder exercises	**Reps**	**Sets**	**Remarks**
Isometric Holds			
Shoulder Press			
Frontal Raise			
Rear Deltoid			
Lateral Raise			
Bicep exercises	**Reps**	**Sets**	**Remarks**
Isometric Hold			
Standing Curls			
Overhead Pull			
Bent over curl			
Triceps exercises	**Reps**	**Sets**	**Remarks**
Overhead press			
Kickbacks			
Overhead push			
Forward press			
Leg exercises	**Reps**	**Sets**	**Remarks**
Squats			
Hip extension			
Hip flexion			
Abd/Adduction			

FIT-BALL
EXERCISES

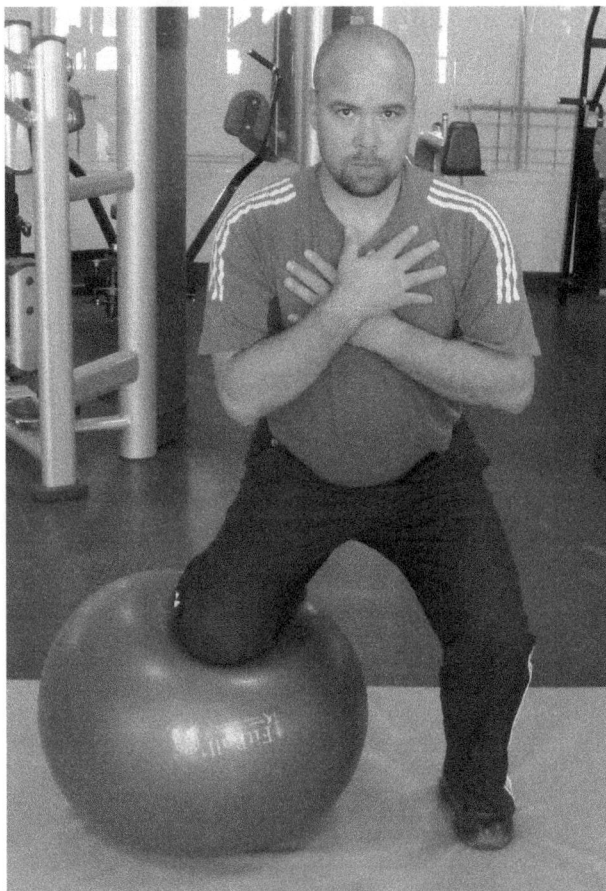

Chapter 5

Back

Exercise 1.1 – Single leg raise

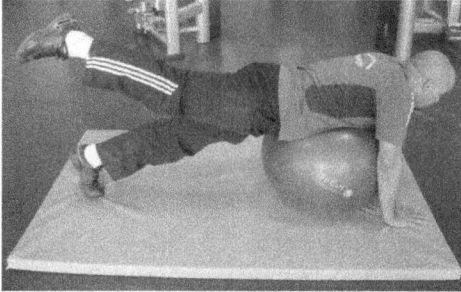

EXERCISE DESCRIPTION

Lie on top of the ball with it positioned around the area of your chest; place your hands on the floor shoulder width apart. Extend your hip above waist height, ensuring at all times that you contract your abdominals whilst breathing out and keep your shoulders as relaxed as possible. Lower your leg to the start position whilst breathing in and repeat, change arms and legs accordingly. This exercise works your glutes in addition to your lower back muscles.

To increase the intensity:

- Do not rest the leg between repetitions;
- Use the same leg until fatigued;
- Hold the leg raised for 2-3 seconds and/or
- Insert a hold midway.

Exercise 1.2 – Alternate arm & leg raise

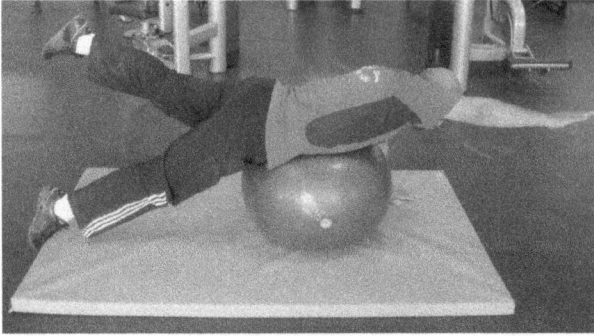

EXERCISE DESCRIPTION

Lie on top of the ball with it positioned around the area of
your chest; place your hands on the floor shoulder width
apart. Extend one of your legs and the opposite arm above
waist height, ensuring at all times that you contract your abdominals whilst breathing out and keep your shoulders as
relaxed as possible. Lower your leg and arm to the start position whilst breathing in and repeat. Change arms and legs
accordingly. This exercise works your glutes and rear deltoid
in addition to your lower back   muscles.

To increase the intensity:

- Do not rest the leg and arm between repetitions;
- Use the same leg until fatigued;
- Hold the leg and arm raised for 2-3 seconds and/or
- Insert a hold midway.

Exercise 1.3 – Ball Pull with knees bent

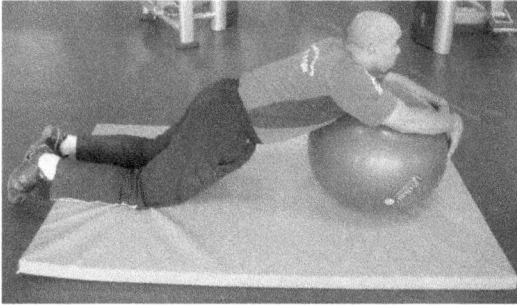

EXERCISE DESCRIPTION

With your knees bent, lean onto the ball with your arms out-stretched around it, Ensuring at all times that you contract your abdominals whilst breathing out and keep your shoulders as relaxed as possible.

The emphasis should be on pulling the ball towards the body and holding for 2-3 seconds, push the ball back to the start position whilst breathing in and repeat.

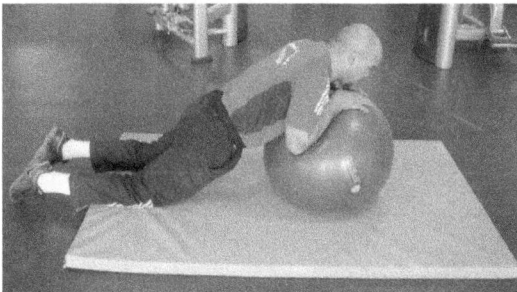

Exercise 1.4 – Ball Pull with straight legs

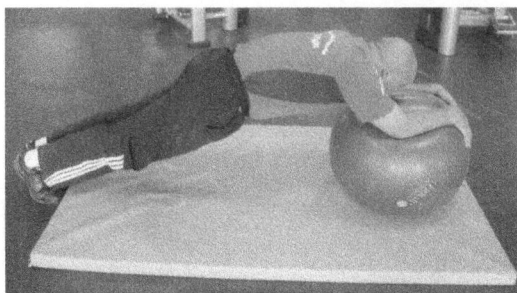

EXERCISE DESCRIPTION

With your legs straight, lean onto the ball with your arms out-stretched around it, Ensuring at all times that you contract your abdominals whilst breathing out and keep your shoulders as relaxed as possible.

The emphasis should be on pulling the ball towards the body and holding for 2-3 seconds, push the ball back to the start position whilst breathing in and repeat.

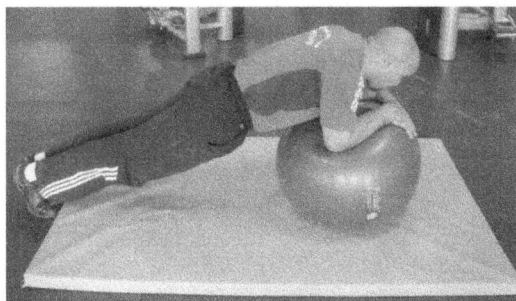

110

Exercise 1.5 – Resistance band reverse flyes

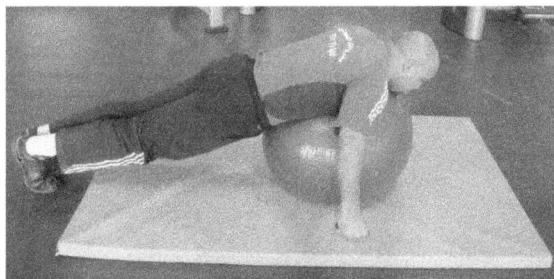

EXERCISE DESCRIPTION

Making sure that the resistance band is not too heavy and positioned securely underneath the centre of the fit-ball. Lie on top of the ball with it positioned around the area of your chest and grasp the band ensuring it is taught enough and that your arms are outstretched to the side with a slight bend at the elbow. Concentrate on bringing your shoulder blades together whilst breathing out and raising your arms above shoulder height.

Ensure at all times that you contract your abdominals whilst breathing out and keep your shoulders as relaxed as possible. Lower the band back to the start position whilst breathing in and repeat.

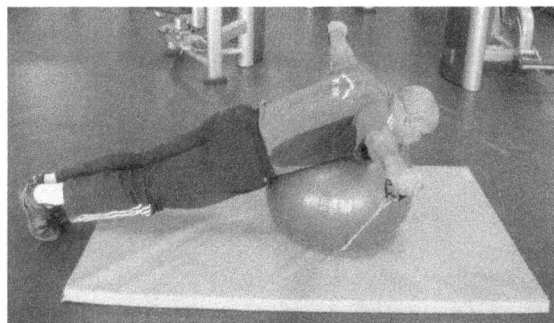

Exercise 1.6 – Dumbbell reverse flyes

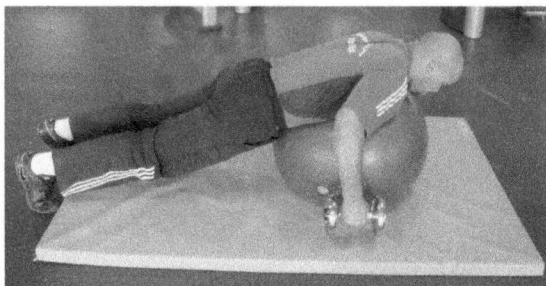

EXERCISE DESCRIPTION

Making sure that the weights are not too heavy and they are positioned close to the centre of the fit-ball. Lie on top of the ball with it positioned around the area of your chest and grasp the dumbbells ensuring that your grip is tight enough and that your arms are outstretched to the side with a slight bend at the elbow. Concentrate on bringing your shoulder blades together whilst breathing out and raising your arms above shoulder height.

Ensure at all times that you contract your abdominals whilst breathing out and keep your shoulders as relaxed as possible. Lower the weights back to the start position whilst breathing in and repeat.

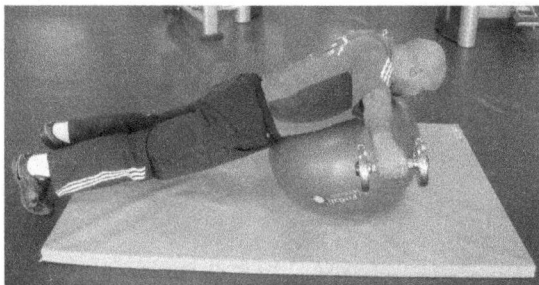

112

Exercise 1.7 – Single arm Dumbbell row

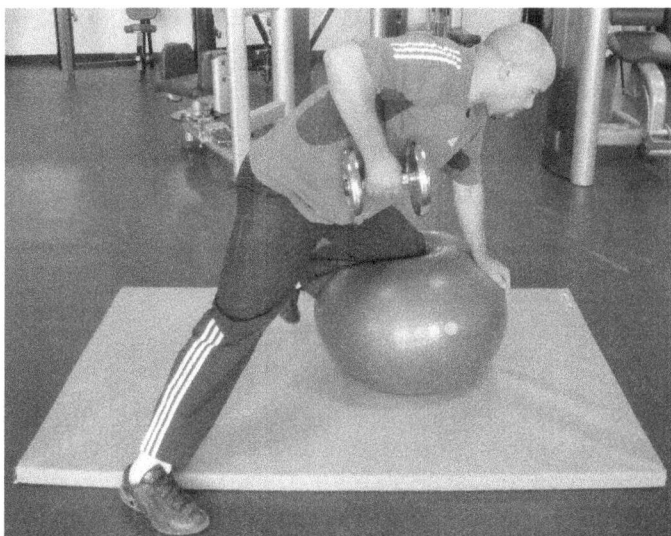

EXERCISE DESCRIPTION

Making sure that the weight is not too heavy and that it is positioned close to the centre of the fit-ball. Kneel on top of the centre of the ball and grasp the dumbbell ensuring that your grip is tight enough and that your arm is straight. Concentrate on using your back muscles only whilst breathing out and bending your arm until the weight is close to the side of your body. Ensure at all times that you contract your abdominals whilst breathing out and keep your shoulders as relaxed as possible.

Lower the weight under control whilst breathing in and repeat accordingly, change arms.

Chest

Exercise 2.1 – Chest Press

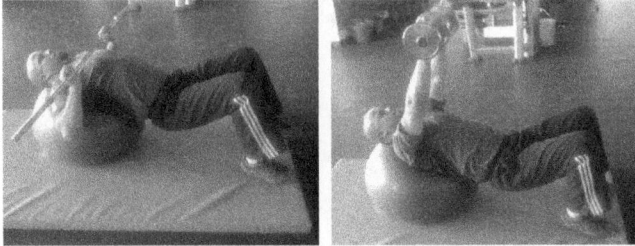

EXERCISE DESCRIPTION

Safety should be your main priority especially when selecting the weight to start with until you have mastered the technique. Position yourself on the fit-ball so that the ball is in the centre of your back. Grip the weight firmly with one or both hands and once you have lifted the weight from the ground you should be positioned correctly on the ball with the weights level with the upper part of your chest and your elbows low where possible. As you breathe out, engage your abdominals and push the weights up whilst straightening your arm(s). Breathe in as you return to the start position and repeat.

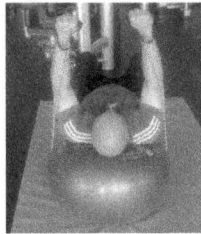

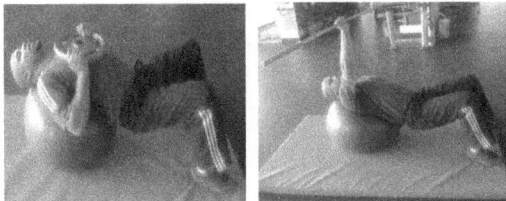

Exercise 2.2 – Flyes

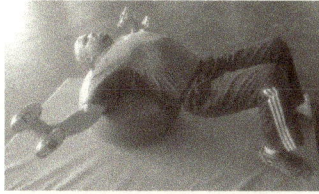

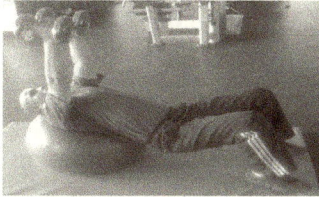

EXERCISE DESCRIPTION

Safety should be your main priority especially when selecting the weight to start with until you have mastered the technique. Position yourself on the fit-ball so that the ball is in the centre of your back. Grip the weight firmly with one or both hands and once you have lifted the weight from the ground you should be positioned correctly on the ball with the weights level with the upper part of your chest and your elbows low where possible but more importantly with your arms outstretched to the side of your body with a slight bend at the elbows. As you breathe out, engage your abdominals and push the weight up with a straight arm(s). Breathe in as you return to the start position and repeat. Your hand position can vary from palms facing towards you or thumbs.

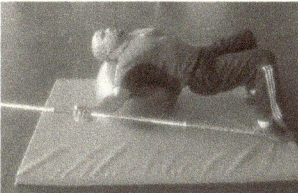

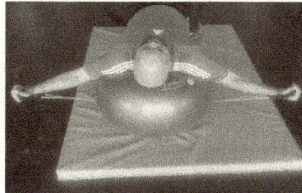

Exercise 2.3 – Pull Over

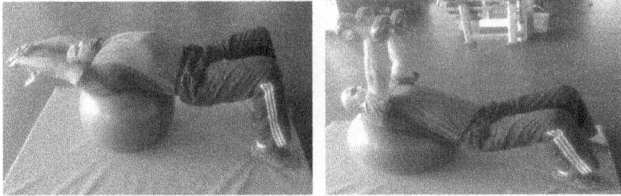

EXERCISE DESCRIPTION

Safety should be your main priority especially when selecting a weight to start with until you have mastered the technique. Position yourself on the fit-ball so that the ball is in the centre of your back. Grip the weight firmly with one or both hands and once you have lifted the weight from the ground you should be positioned correctly on the ball with your arm(s) above your head and as you breathe out, engage your abdominals and pull the weight towards your lower chest. Your arm(s) should remain as straight as is comfortable, breathe in as you return to the start position and repeat.

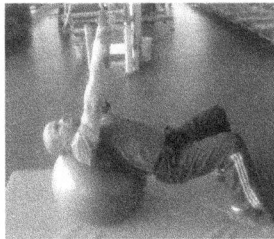

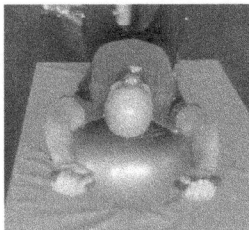

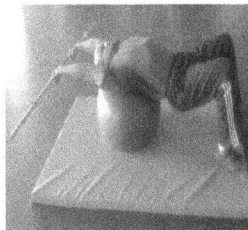

Exercise 2.4 – Push Up

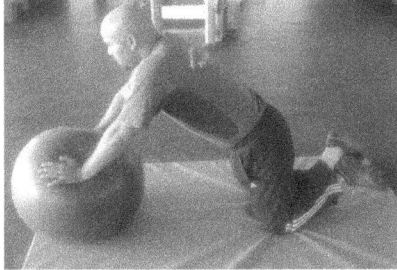

EXERCISE DESCRIPTION

From the kneeling position ensure that your hands are level with your shoulders and that you lean onto the fit-ball. Your shoulders should be relaxed and your hips and shoulders should remain facing towards the ground along with your head and eyes. Initiate the movement from the abdominals and lower your upper body until your chest is close to the ball whilst breathing in. Breathe out as you raise your upper body back to the start position. As you tire, concentrate on your breathing whilst compressing your abdominals and lower back; tense your whole body (not shoulders) to assist you in keeping good form. If this is too easy you can begin by making it more difficult by replacing your knees with your feet i.e. in the full push up position. Maintaining control throughout the movement is important whilst breathing correctly.

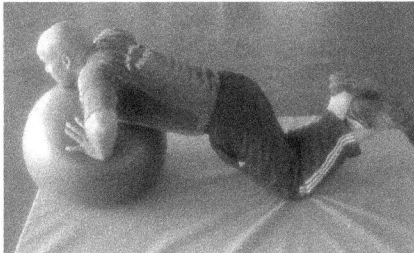

Shoulders

Exercise 3.1 – Isometric Holds

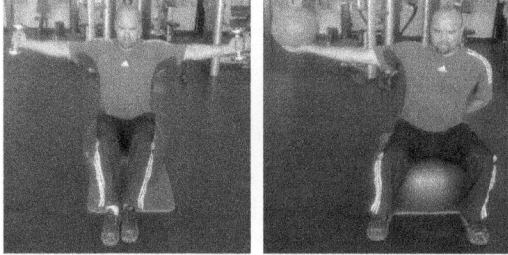

EXERCISE DESCRIPTION

Whichever hold you are doing you must ensure that wherever possible your posture is good i.e. maintaining body alignment with your head, eyes, shoulders and hips inline and facing forwards as much as possible. Your abdominals should be initiated prior and during each hold with your shoulders relaxed as much as possible. All of the above movements are explained in the exercises to follow; therefore all you are doing is mimicking those muscle actions and placing a hold within the ranges, your breathing should remain controlled and should not be forced.

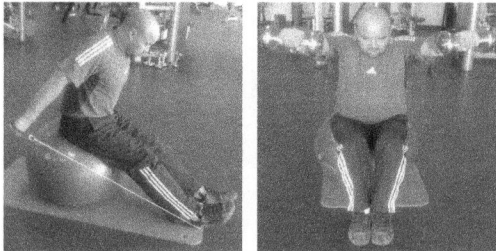

Exercise 3.2 – Shoulder Press

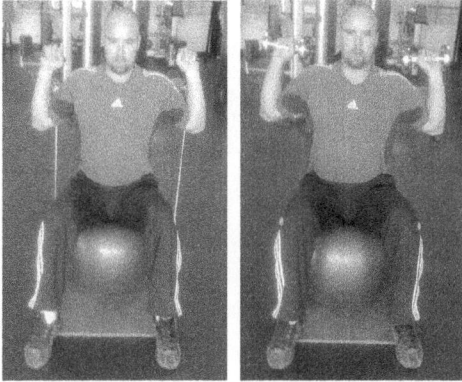

EXERCISE DESCRIPTION

Select a safe weight to start with until you have mastered the technique and position yourself on the fit-ball with your feet flat on the floor and level. Grip the weights firmly with one or both hands and position your hand(s) just above the height of your shoulder(s) with your elbow(s) low and close to the side of your body. As you breathe out, engage your abdominals and raise the resistance up and above your head with your arms outstretched and hold, breathe in as you return to the start position and repeat

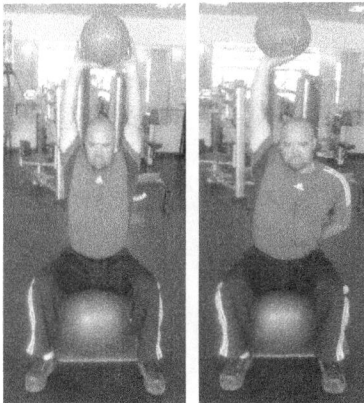

Exercise 3.3 – Frontal Raise

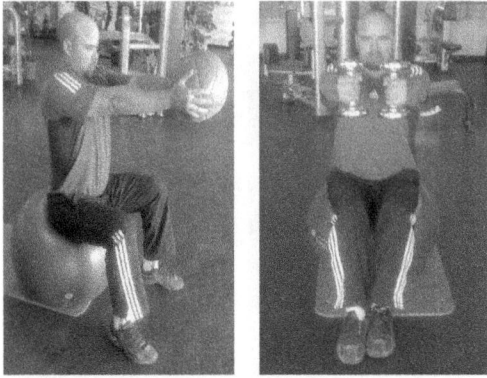

EXERCISE DESCRIPTION

Select a safe weight to start with until you have mastered the technique and position yourself on the fit-ball with your feet flat on the floor and level. Grip the weights firmly with both hands and initially they should be positioned down and close to the front of the body with both arms straight. As you breathe out, engage your abdominals and raise the weights up and level with your shoulders and hold. Attempt to keep them level, along with keeping your arm straight, albeit with a very slight bend at the elbow to avoid injury. Keep your shoulders relaxed and breathe in as you return to the start position and repeat.

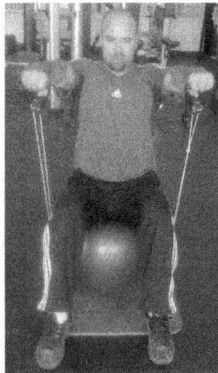

Exercise 3.4 – Lateral Raise

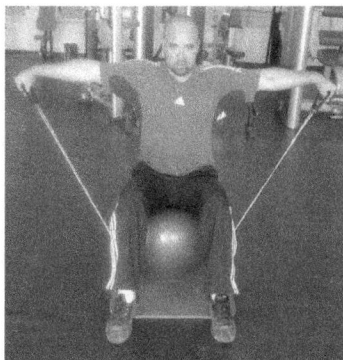

EXERCISE DESCRIPTION

Select a safe weight to start with until you have mastered the technique and position yourself on the fit-ball with your feet flat on the floor and level. Grip the weights firmly with both hands and initially they should be positioned down and close to the side of the body with both arms straight. As you breathe out, engage your abdominals and raise the weights out to the side and level with your shoulders and hold. Attempt to keep them level, along with keeping your arm straight, albeit with a very slight bend at the elbow to avoid injury. Breathe in as you return to the start position and repeat.

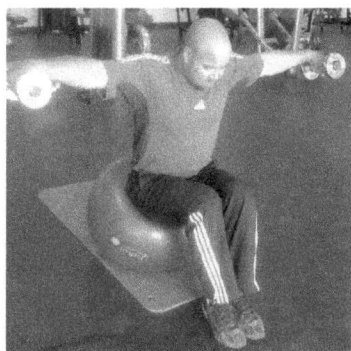

Exercise 3.5 – Prone lying raises

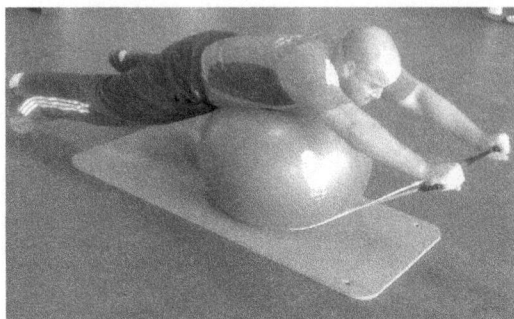

EXERCISE DESCRIPTION

Select a safe resistance to start with until you have mastered the technique and position yourself lying on the ball with your legs in a stable position for balance but level. Grip the bands firmly with both hands and initially they should be positioned down and close to the ball with both arms relaxed. As you breathe out, engage your abdominals and raise the bands up level with your shoulders and beyond if possible and hold. Attempt to keep the bands level along with keeping your arms straight albeit with a very slight bend at the elbow to avoid injury. Breathe in as you return to the start position and repeat. Advance with your feet as you get more confident (read intro)

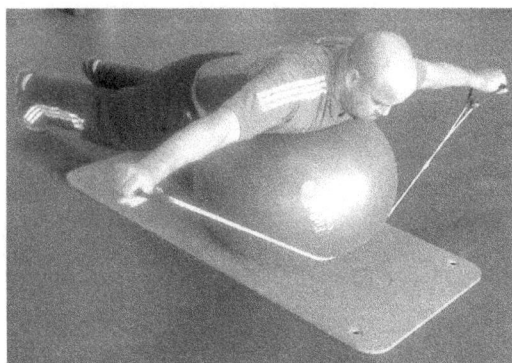

Exercise 3.6 – Fit-ball Caterpillar

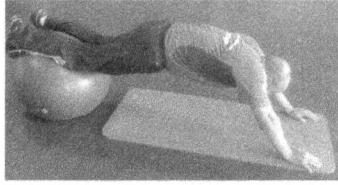

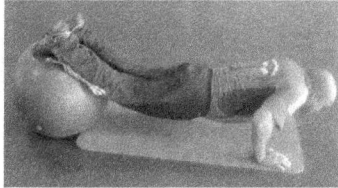

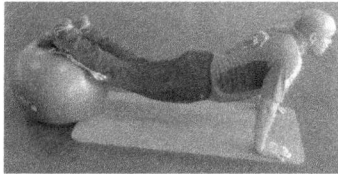

EXERCISE DESCRIPTION

With your feet on the ball, your hands level on the floor and around shoulder width apart, hold your body in a V position as best you can with your backside raised up slightly. Throughout all 3 movements your abdominals should be initiated and as you breathe out you should roll your bodyweight forwards using only your shoulders, roll down and forwards bending your arms at the elbows until your chest almost brushes the ground and then roll upwards straightening your arms and hold. Breathe in until you reverse the movement by rolling your shoulders in the opposite direction until you are back in the start position. Repeat the movement but keep the shoulders pulled down and backwards as much as possible which will ensure that your upper spine and head are relaxed and not under too much tension.

Biceps

Exercise 4.1 – Isometric Holds

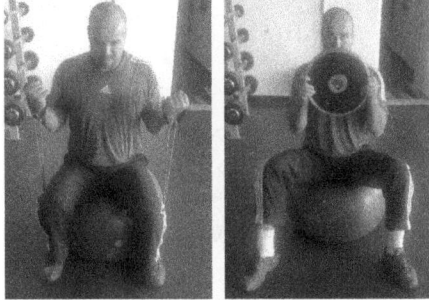

EXERCISE DESCRIPTION

Select a safe resistance/weight to start with until you have mastered the technique and position yourself in the seated position on a fit-ball with your legs in a balanced position and level. Grip the bands/weight(s) firmly with one or both hand(s) and positioned down and close to the body with straight arms. As you breathe out, engage your abdominals and raise the resistance/weight(s) up by bending your elbows and hold. Attempt to hold for a challenging length of time and then breathe in as you slowly return to the start position and repeat. Attempt to vary the exercise by completing a single or double arm hold.

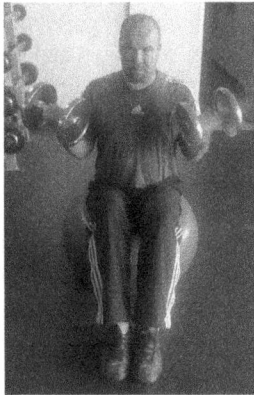

Exercise 4.2 – Resistance band curls

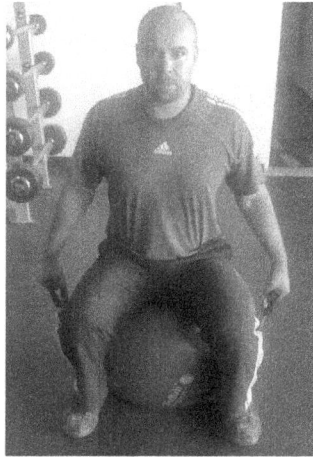

EXERCISE DESCRIPTION

Select a safe resistance to start with until you have mastered the technique and position yourself in the seated position on a fit-ball with your legs in a balanced position and level. Grip the bands firmly with both hands and positioned down and close to the side of your body with straight arms. As you breathe out, engage your abdominals and raise the bands up by bending your elbows and hold. Attempt to keep the bands level and breathe in as you slowly return to the start position and repeat. Attempt to vary the exercise by completing a single or double arm curl.

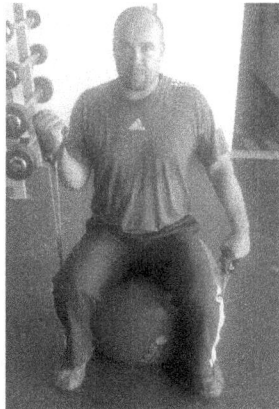

Exercise 4.3 – Hammer Curls

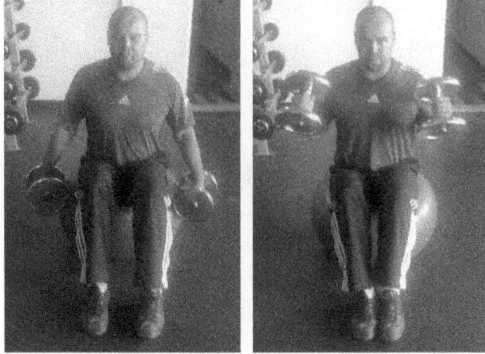

EXERCISE DESCRIPTION

Select a safe weight to start with until you have mastered the technique and position yourself in the seated position on a fit-ball with your legs in a balanced position and level. Grip the weights firmly with both hands (knuckles facing outwards) and positioned down and close to the side of your body with straight arms. As you breathe out, engage your abdominals and raise the dumbbells up fully by bending your elbows and hold. Attempt to keep the weights level and breathe in as you slowly return to the start position and repeat. Attempt to vary the exercise by completing a single or double arm curl (picture below).

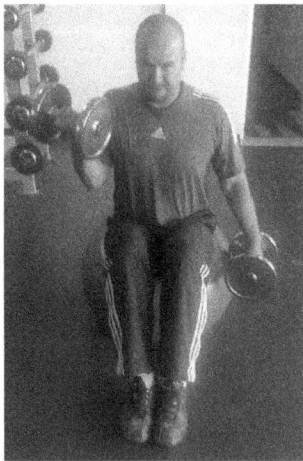

Exercise 4.4 – Variation of Curls

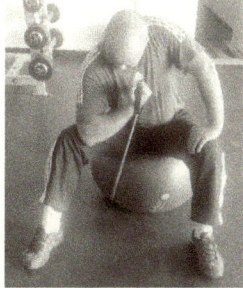

EXERCISE DESCRIPTION

Whichever weight/resistance you use it should be safe enough to start with until you have mastered the technique and position yourself in the seated position on a fit-ball with your legs in a balanced position and level. Grip the resistance/ weight(s) firmly with one or both hands and positioned down with straight arms. As you breathe out, engage your abdominals and raise the resistance/weight(s) up fully by bending your elbows and hold. Attempt to keep the band(s)/weight(s) level and breathe in as you slowly return to the start position and repeat. Attempt to vary the exercise by completing a single or double arm curl (picture below).

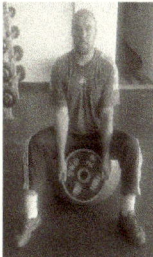

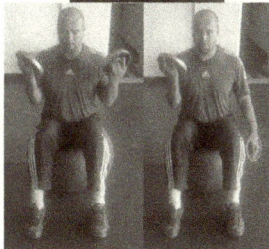

Triceps

Exercise 5.1 – Dumbbell overhead press (Back lying)

Both arms   **Single arm**

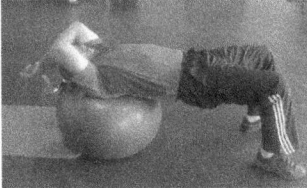 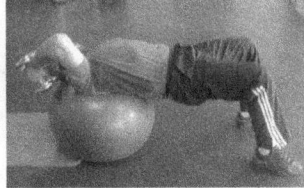

EXERCISE DESCRIPTION

Select a safe weight to start with until you have mastered the technique and position yourself lying flat on the fit-ball with your arms straight and above your head. Breathe in and bend your arms at the elbow lowering the weight down whilst attempting to keep your elbows as close together as you can without moving the remainder of your arm. Initiate the abdominals as you breathe out and raise the weight back to the start position whilst contracting your triceps as you straighten the arms. As you get more confident move your feet closer together but keep your hips high at all times. Also, try single arm once you have perfected the technique with both.

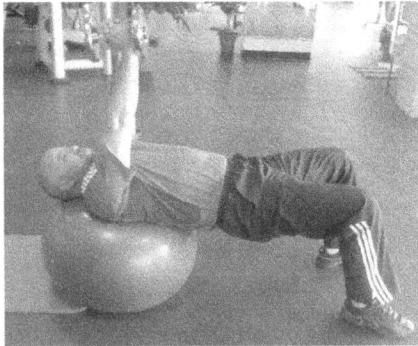

Exercise 5.2 – Barbell overhead press

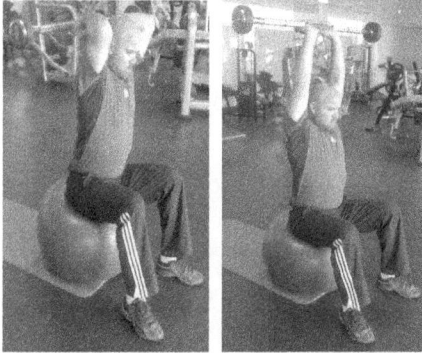

EXERCISE DESCRIPTION

Select a safe weight to start with until you have mastered the technique and position yourself sat or lying on the fit-ball. Start with your arms straight above your head with your hands close together and equal distance from the centre of the bar. Breathe in and bend your arms at the elbow lowering the weight down behind you whilst attempting to keep your elbow as close together as you can without moving the remainder of your arms. Initiate the abdominals as you breathe out and raise the weight back to the start position whilst contracting your triceps as you straighten the arms, repeat the movement. As you get more confident move your feet closer together and if lying on the fit-ball keep your hips high at all times.

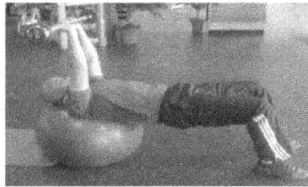

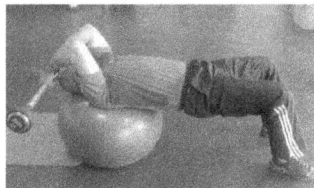

Exercise 5.3 – Kickbacks

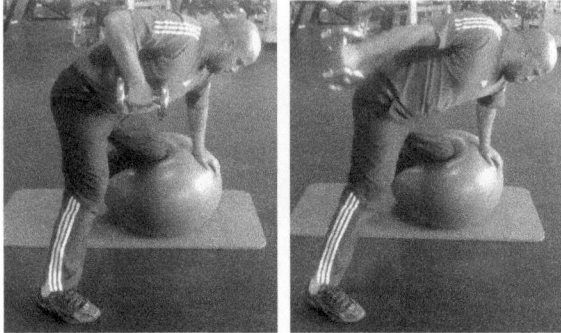

EXERCISE DESCRIPTION

Select a safe weight to start with until you have mastered the technique and position yourself knelt on a fit-ball with your back straight and perpendicular to the bench. Start with one arm resting on the fit-ball (for stability) and the other arm bent at the elbow with the weight/band close to the body. Breathe out as you straighten the arm behind you whilst contracting your triceps, breathe in as you return the weight/band back to the start position and change arms as you repeat the movement. As you get more confident take your hand away from the fit-ball and/or move your leg closer to the ball.

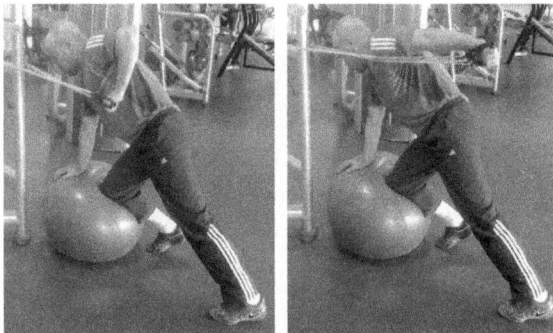

Exercise 5.4 – Close arm press

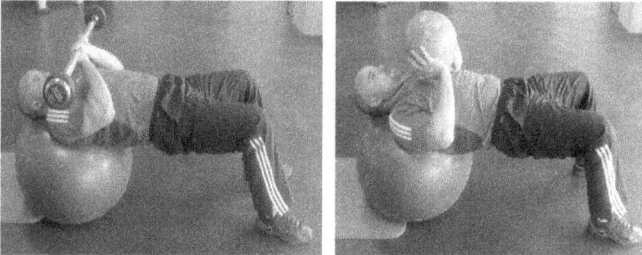

EXERCISE DESCRIPTION

Select a safe weight to start with until you have mastered the technique and position yourself lying flat on a fit-ball with your hands positioned close together but equal distance from the centre of the weighted object. Start with the weight close to your chest; initiate the abdominals as you breathe out and raise the object up as you straighten your arms to contract your triceps. Breathe in as you lower the object back to the start position and repeat the movement. As you get more confident move your feet closer together and keep your hips high at all times.

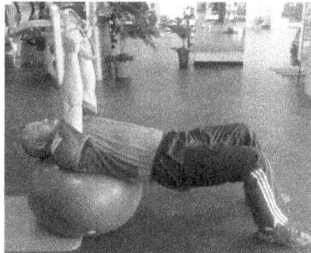

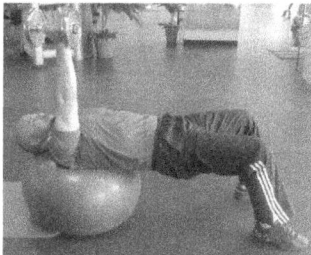

Exercise 5.5 – Other variations

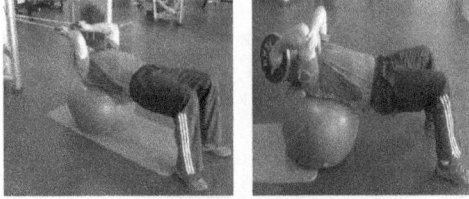

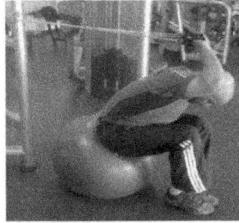

EXERCISE DESCRIPTION

Select a safe weight to start with until you have mastered the technique and position yourself sat or lying on the fit-ball. Whichever exercise you are completing make sure that you start by breathing in whilst bending your arms at the elbow lowering the weight down behind you whilst attempting to keep your elbow as close together as you can without moving the remainder of your arms. Initiate the abdominals as you breathe out and raise the weight back to the start position whilst contracting your triceps as you straighten the arms, re-peat the movement. As you get more confident move your feet closer together and if lying on the fit-ball keep your hips high at all times.

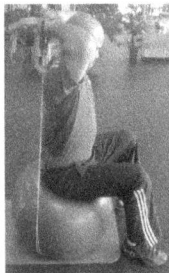

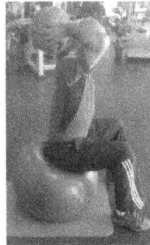

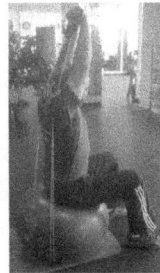

Legs

Exercise 6.1 – Hip Flexors

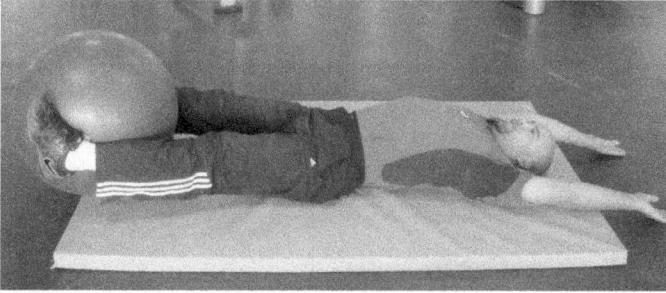

EXERCISE DESCRIPTION

Lying on your back, place the ball in between your legs, squeeze the ball with your legs and raise your legs up and in-line with your hips. Ensure at all times that you contract your abdominals and press the small of your back towards the ground whilst breathing out. Lower your legs under control whilst breathing in and repeat accordingly. Your aim should be to keep the legs from touching the floor and to apply a 3-5 second hold whilst keeping the legs as straight as possible.

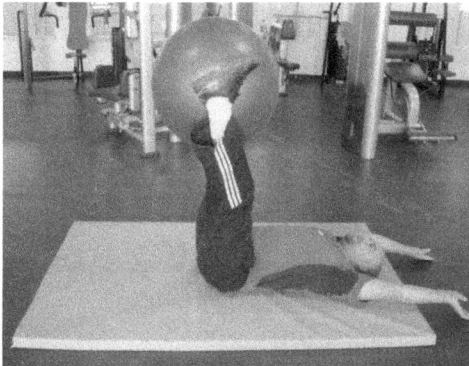

Exercise 6.2 – Leg Bridge

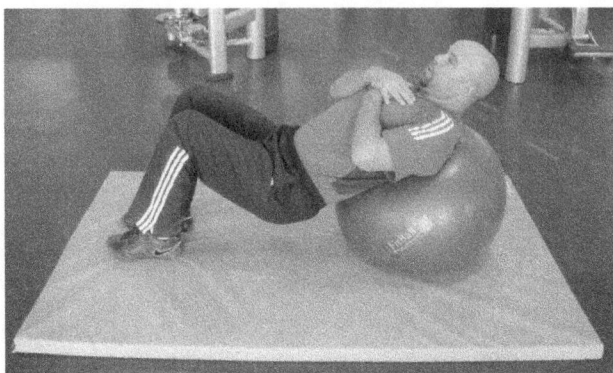

EXERCISE DESCRIPTION

Lie on the ball with your arms outstretched (at first) and place your feet firmly on the floor (not too close together) initiate the movement from the abdominals and raise your hips until they are inline with the shoulders and tops of the knees, breathe out and hold for 3-5 seconds. Return to the start position whilst breathing in and repeat the exercise, progress accordingly with the arms.

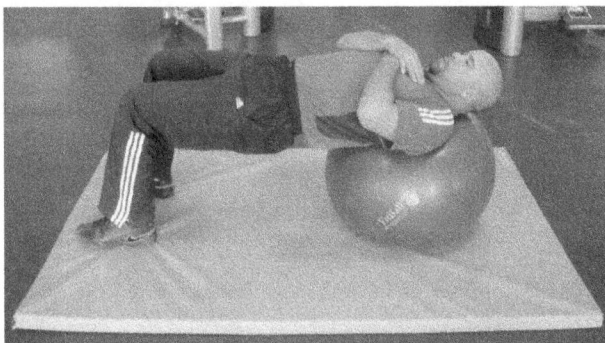

Exercise 6.3 – Abductor/Adductor

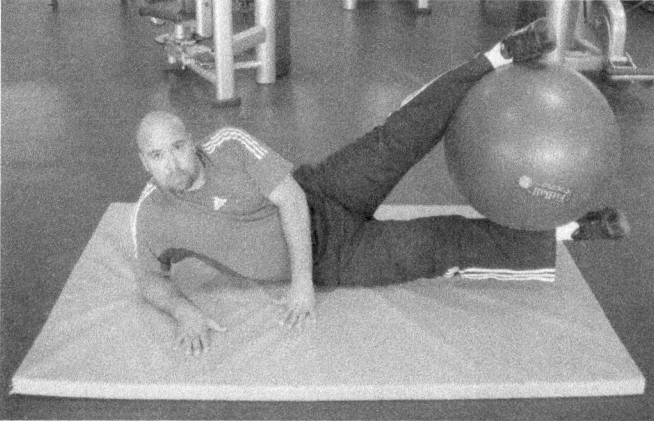

EXERCISE DESCRIPTION

Lie on your side with your body as straight as possible, keeping the ball squeezed between your feet. Raise your legs as high off the ground as you can without twisting the body, whilst breathing out and return back to the start position whilst breathing in. Your aim should be to keep the legs from touching the floor and to apply a 3-5 second hold whilst keeping the legs as straight as possible. You must initiate the movement from the abdominals and try not to use your upper body too much, relax the shoulders at all times.

Exercise 6.4 – Wall Squat

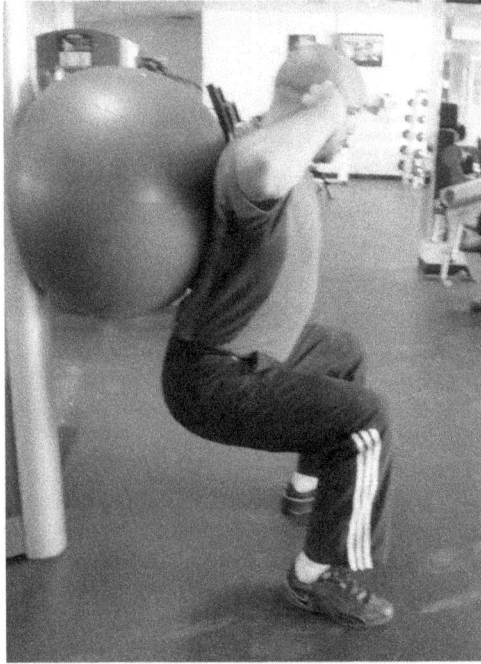

EXERCISE DESCRIPTION

Place the ball behind you and position your feet shoulder
width apart, relax the head and shoulders. Lower your body
until your legs are at a 90 degree angle whilst breathing out.
Return to the start position whilst breathing in ensuring that
your legs are straight and the ball remains just above the small
of the back. Your feet should be level and so use a line for
guidance, your knees should also be behind your toes at all
times.

Exercise 6.5 – Single Leg Squat

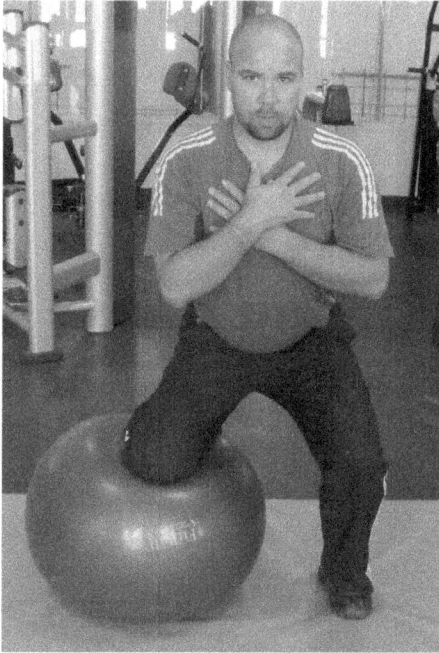

EXERCISE DESCRIPTION

Place one knee on the ball with the other flat on the floor, re-lax the head and shoulders. Lower your body until your leg is at a 90 degree angle whilst breathing out. Return to the start position whilst breathing in ensuring that your leg is straight and the ball remains as still as possible. You should endeavour to keep your knee behind your toe at all times, change legs accordingly.

Fit-ball program – (template)

Back exercises	Reps	Sets	Remarks
Alt arm & leg raise			
Ball Pull bent & straight legs			
Res-band rev flyes			
Db reverse flyes			
Single arm Db row			
Chest exercises	**Reps**	**Sets**	**Remarks**
Chest Press			
Flyes			
Pull Over			
Push Up			
Shoulder exercises	**Reps**	**Sets**	**Remarks**
Isometric Holds			
Shoulder Press			
Frontal Raise			
Prone lying raises			
Fit-ball Caterpillar			
Bicep exercises	**Reps**	**Sets**	**Remarks**
Isometric Holds			
Resistance band curls			
Hammer Curls			
Variation of Curls			
Triceps exercises	**Reps**	**Sets**	**Remarks**
Dumbbell overhead press (Back lying)			
B-bell overhead press			
Kickbacks			
Close arm press			
Other variations			
Leg exercises	**Reps**	**Sets**	**Remarks**
Hip Flexors			
Leg Bridge			
Abductor/Adductor			
Wall Squat			
Single Leg Squat			

GET YOUR OWN SIX PACK

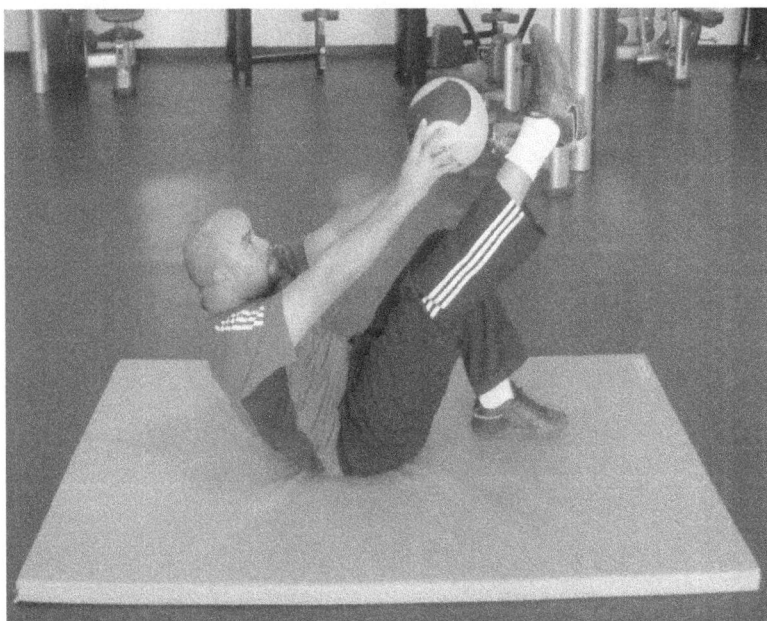

Chapter 6

Abdominal exercises:

Thousands if not millions of gym users often wonder why it is so difficult to get a six pack. The actual processes of getting a six pack are quite straight forward and at the same time nothing that you probably haven't already heard before. When it comes to your abs it requires only that you decrease your intake of Fatty foods and of course certain exercises done correctly. Everything that you do fitness wise should be initiated by the power of your abdominals, from standing up straight, walking or any exercise, especially with weights.

Aim:

The aim of this workbook is to give you a large selection (library) of exercises so that you can select one's that work best for you.

Intensity levels:

High intensity interval training (H.I.I.T) should accompany the exercises in this workbook. As with all exercises you should aim to control all movements i.e. whatever the exercise, it should be completed slowly during the concentric and eccentric aspects (up & down). The abdominals should be initiated prior & during every exercise and this way you will work them 100%. The position of your feet & arms whilst on the fit-ball is also very vital to your results i.e. hands out to the side takes less control of your abdominals than your hands across your chest. The closer together your feet are, the more balance is required; try this out as you master the technique on the fit-ball for each exercise.

How much is enough:

As always, use a diary to write down what you can achieve in the time you have, you can start off by doing each exercise to a certain amount of reps or to a set time, so long as you control each movement. Stay out of your comfort zone and don't just do the exercises you find easy…always test your body and keep it thinking about what is coming next!!! The more difficult you find a certain exercise you can guarantee that it is that exercise that will get you the better results.

Posture & Breathing:

You should retain good posture throughout any exercise i.e. your head, shoulders and hips should be inline & facing forwards at all times. This should not change irrespective of which position you are in, whether it is standing, sitting, on your back or on your front. It is advised that you breathe out during any exertion to avoid any health issues. It is extremely important that the abdominals are initiated first, before all movements.

Important notes: Some people believe that you have to do 1000's of sit ups to get results. With a healthy diet and a reduction in body fat alongside controlled exercises that require you to focus, you will achieve the results you require.

Before attempting any exercise you must always see your doctor before exercising, especially if you have any existing injuries or conditions.

Certain exercises within this chapter cannot be done at home but are included as extra information.

Beginner Abdominal Exercises

Exercise 1.1 – Bent knee Sit Up (arms across chest)

Start Position:

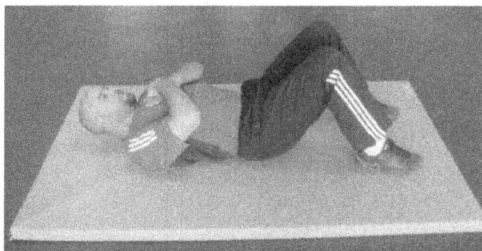

Variation of exercises:

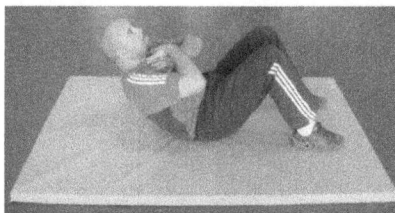

A: Raise your shoulders off the ground using the abdominals only

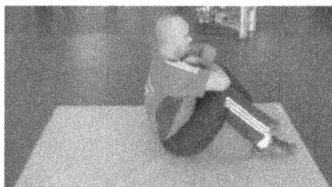

B: Raise your back off the ground using the abdominals only

Exercise 1.2 – Leg Raises (arms by side)

Start Position: Endeavour to keep your feet off the ground

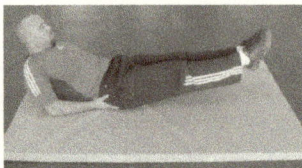

Choice of Exercises:

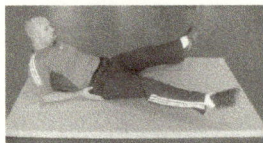

A: open/close your legs to the side

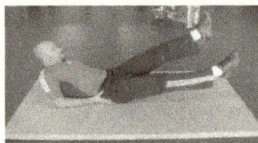

B: up and down

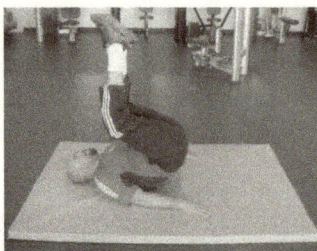

C: Raise your hips off the ground using the abdominals only

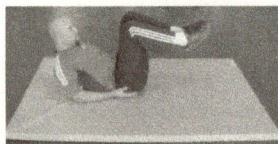

D: Raise your knees to your chest

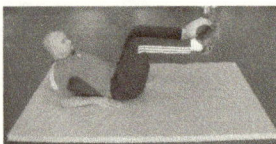

E: Add a weight

Exercise 1.3 - Sit Ups (arms above head)

Start Position:

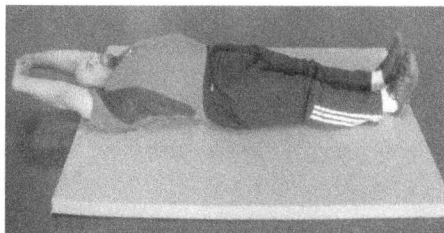

Choice of Exercises:

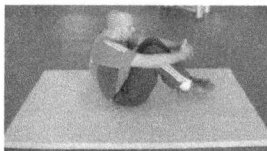

A: Sit up to grasp your bent knees

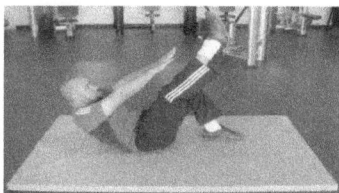

B: Sit up to touch the ankle of one straight leg

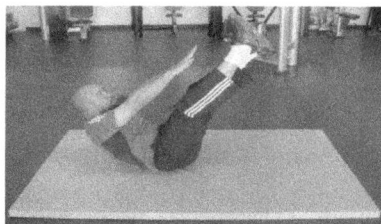

C: Sit up and hold with 2 straight legs

Exercise 1.4 - Sit Ups (hands on head)

Start Position: On your back or on your side

Choice of Exercises:

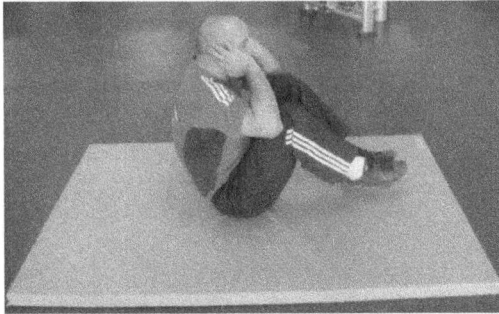

A: Sit up to touch the knees with your elbows

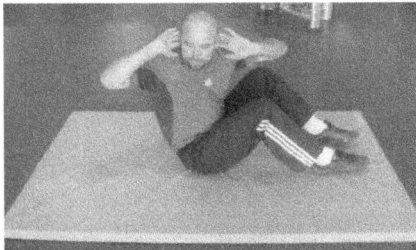

B: Sit up to touch the knee with the opposing elbow

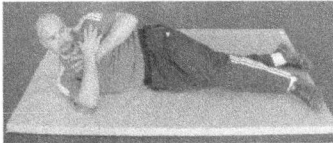

C: Sit up to the side and hold (hands across chest)

146

Exercise 1.5 – Beginner Sit Ups (utilising a fit-ball)

Start Position: Sat on the ball, legs on the ball or between your feet

Choice of Exercises:

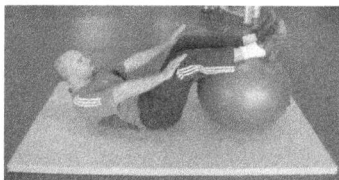

A: Sit up to touch the knees with your finger tips

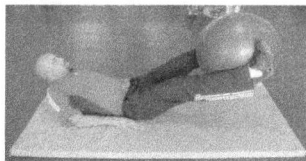

B: Raise the ball towards your hips with legs bent

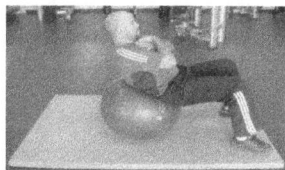

C: Sit up slowly and hold

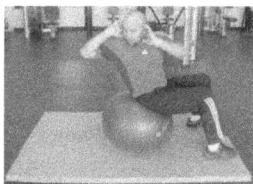

D: Sit up slowly and twist

Exercise 1.6 – Beginner Machines

Starting out: Always consult a personal trainer or gym instructor first

Choice of Exercises:

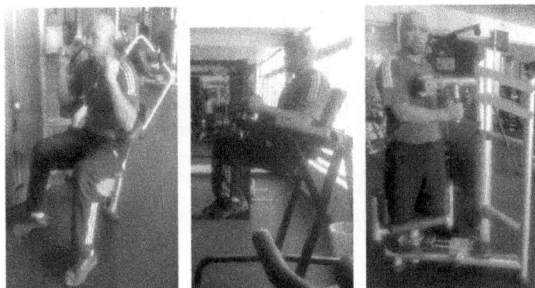

A: Crunch, twist and raise the knees to chest height

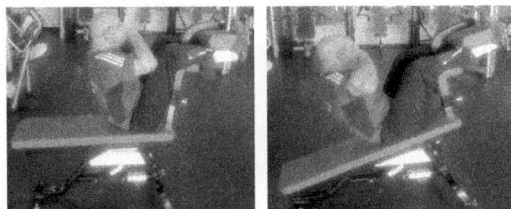

B: Fix the legs and curl up and down slowly

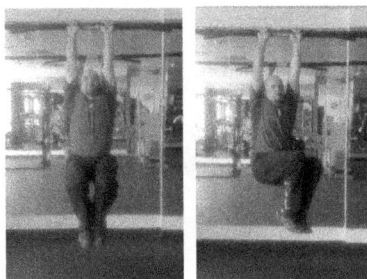

C: Ensure your grip is tight; raise the knees to waist height and / or twist to work your obliques.

148

Intermediate Abdominal Exercises

Exercise 2.1 – Weighted ball in hands

Start positions: Ball in your outstretched arms

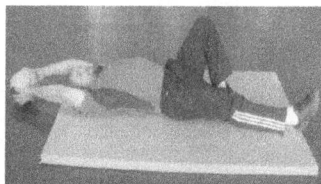

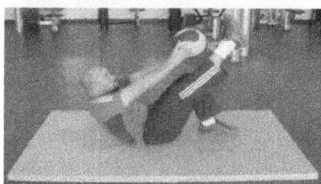

A: With 1 leg bent curl up, touch your other leg with the ball

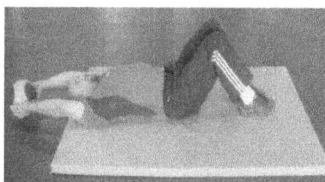

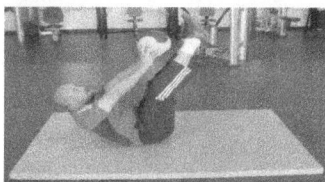

B: With both legs bent curl up, touch both your legs with the ball

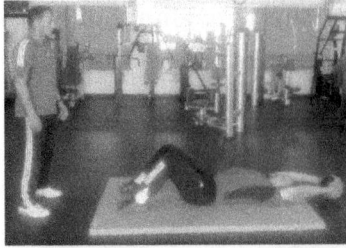

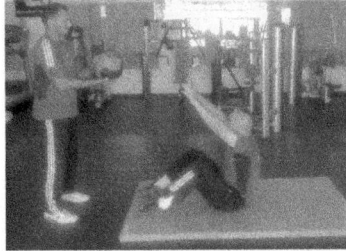

C: With both legs bent, keep ball above head as long as possible with arms straight, curl up, breathe out and throw at the wall - or to someone.

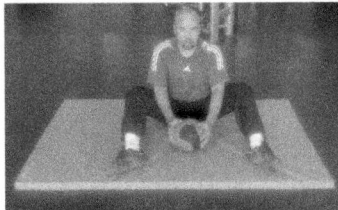

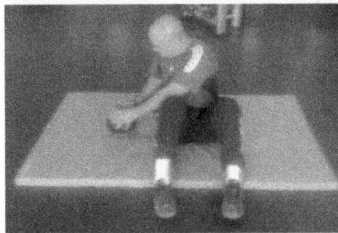

D: Twist at the waist and touch the ball down behind you, repeat to opposite side.

Exercise 2.2 – Weighted ball in feet

Starting out: Keep your feet off the ground at all times

Choice of Exercises:

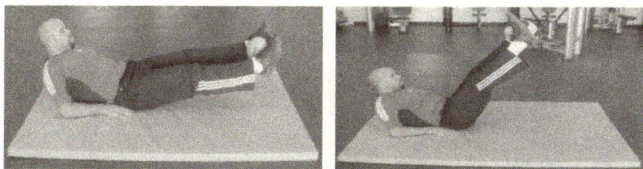

A: Raise your legs from the floor, hold, lower and raise.

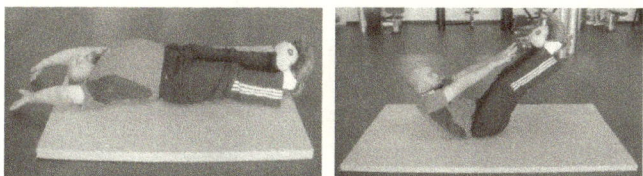

B: With both legs straight, curl up, touch the ball with both hands & slowly lower

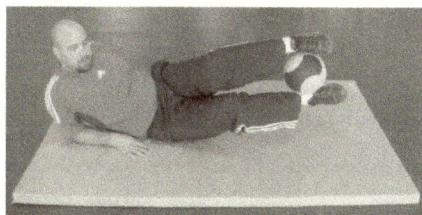

C: Twist at the waist; touch your knees down to each side, repeat to other side

151

Exercise 2.3 – Partner Exercises

Choice of Exercises:

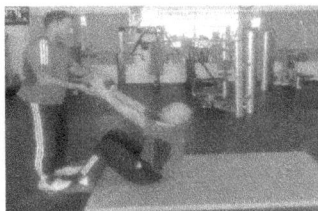

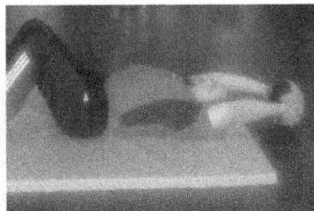

A: With both legs bent, keep ball above head for as long as possible with arms straight, curl up, breathe out and pass the ball to your partner

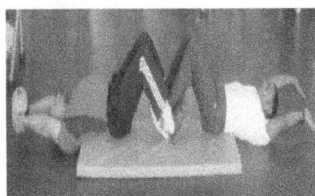

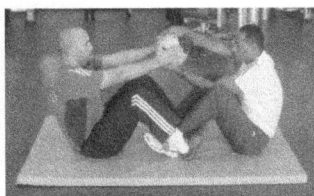

B: With both legs bent, curl up & pass the ball to your partner

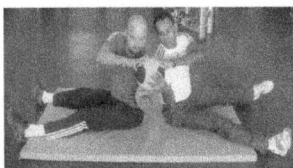

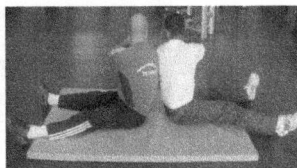

C: Twist at the waist; pass the ball to your partner, repeat to other side

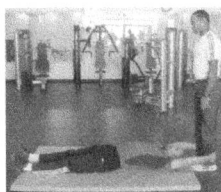

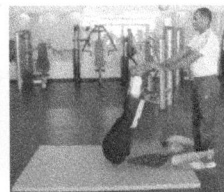

D: Contract your abs, raise your legs towards your partner and breathe out

Exercise 2.4 – Intermediate Abs (utilising a fit-ball)

Choice of Exercises:

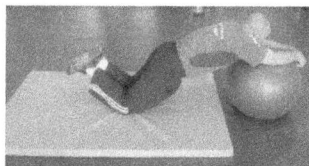

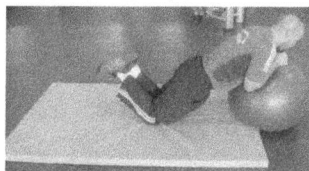

A: With both knees resting, lean on the ball with your arms outstretched, pull the ball towards you as you breathe out and without moving at the waist

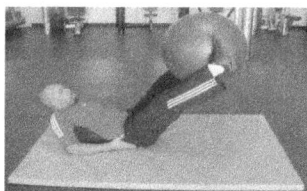

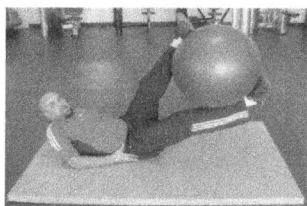

B: With both legs straight, keep the ball in between your feet & twist at the waist

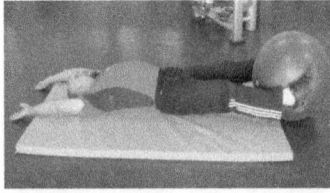

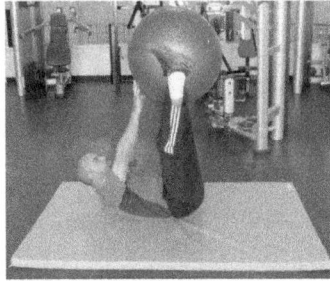

C: Raise both your upper & lower body whilst breathing out, touch the ball

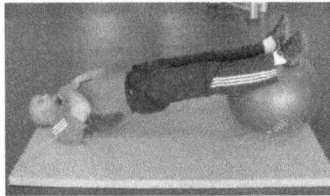

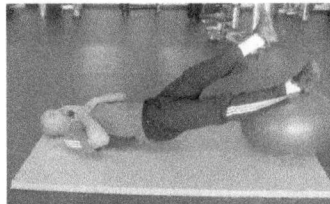

D: With just your shoulders on the floor, press down on the ball with one leg, whilst raising the other, trying to keep your hips high at all times

Advanced Abdominal Exercises

Exercise 3.1 – Bodyweight with minimum equipment

Choice of Exercises:

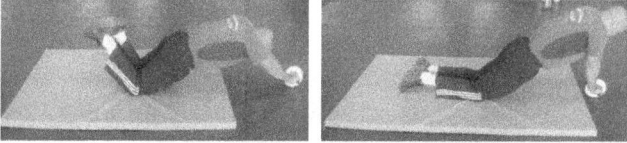

A: With both knees resting, lean on the wheel with your arms outstretched, push & pull the wheel without moving at the waist, Progress to feet on floor

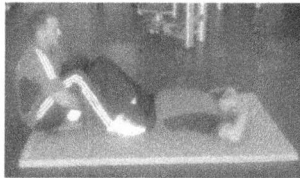

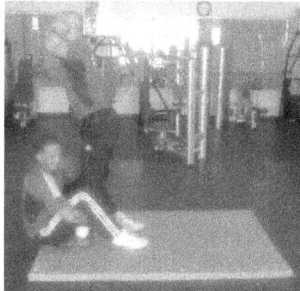

B: Stand up from lying on your back, with or without a partner

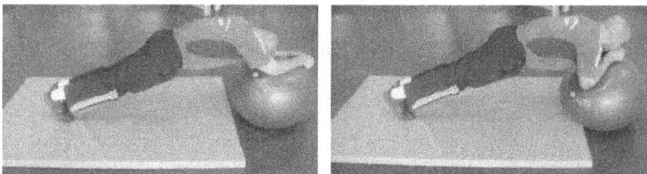

C: With both feet on the floor with your arms outstretched, pull the ball towards you as you breathe out and without moving at the waist

Exercise 3.2 – Advanced Abs (utilising machines)

Choice of Exercises:

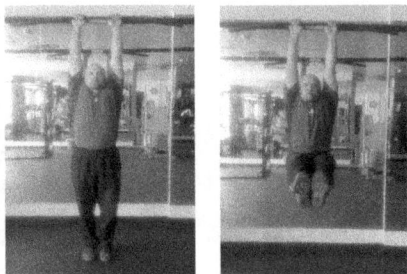

A: Ensure your grip is tight; raise the legs to waist whilst breathing out

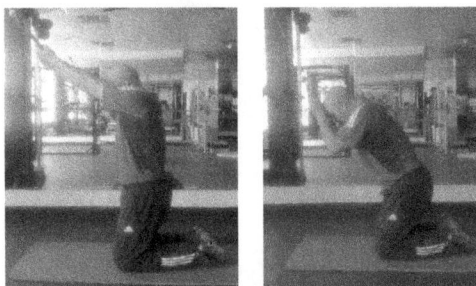

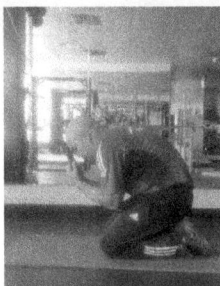

B: Pull cable or rope whilst contracting your abdominals & breathing out

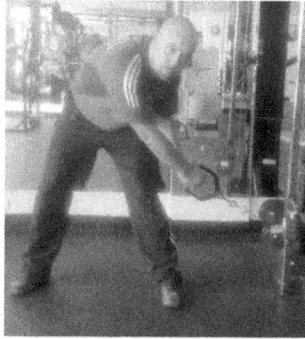

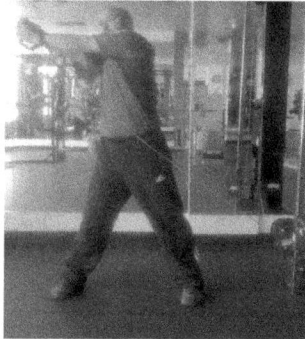

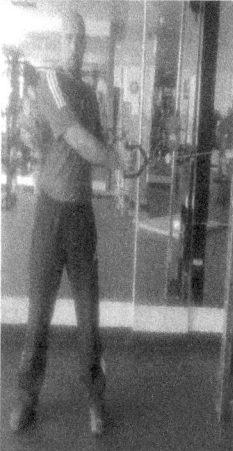

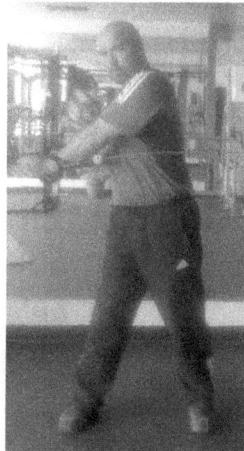

C: Pull the cable up or down dependant on setting, also pull from the side & twist, initiate the abdominals/obliques in order to pull the cable, not the arms.

Exercise 3.3 – Advanced Abs (utilising barbell)

Choice of Exercises:

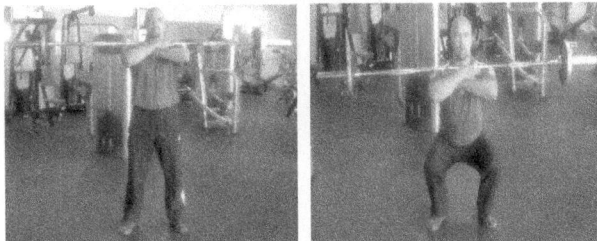

A: Squat down & up under the sole control of your abdominals, control breathing

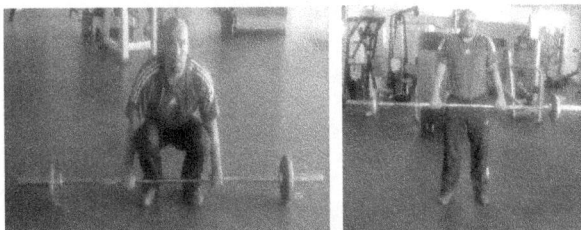

B: Stand up & raise your shoulders utilising your abdominals, whilst breathing out

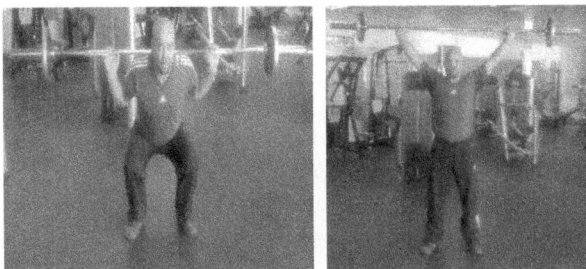

C: Stand up & raise the bar up above your head, utilising your abdominals, whilst breathing out.

158

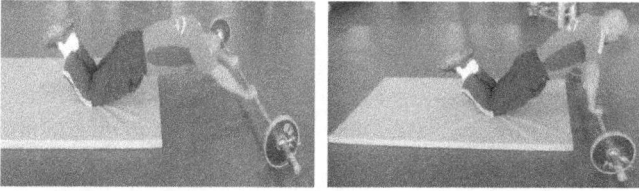

D: With both knees on the floor with your arms outstretched, pull the ball towards you as you breathe out, without moving at the waist. Progress to feet on the floor

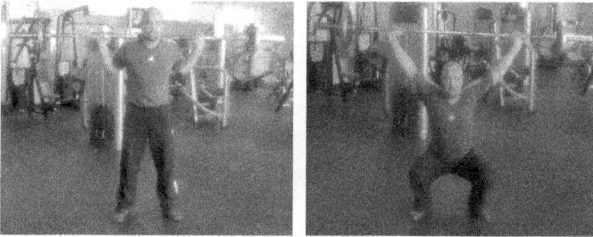

E: Squat down under the sole control of your abdominals, raise the bar up above your head whilst breathing out. Breathe in as you stand up and lower the bar

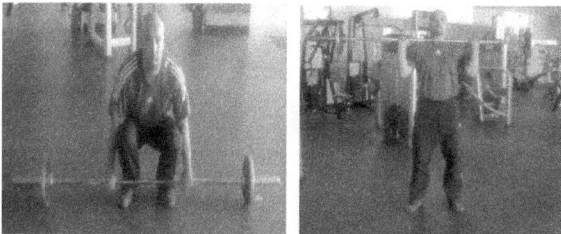

(1)

(2)

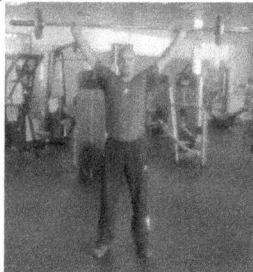

(3)

F: Stand up & raise the bar to your shoulders & then above your head whilst breathing out. Attempt to do this at speed whilst using your abdominals.

159

Exercise 3.4 – Advanced Abs (utilising dumbbells)

Choice of Exercises:

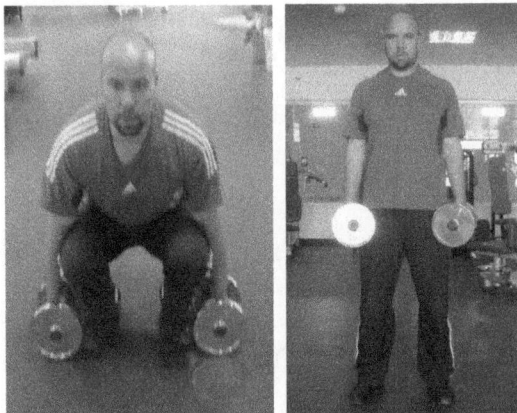

A: Stand up utilising your abdominals, whilst breathing out

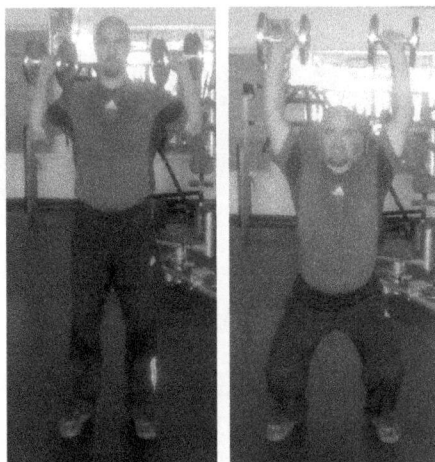

B: Squat down under control of your abs, raise the dumbbells above your head whilst breathing out. Breathe in as you stand up & lower them

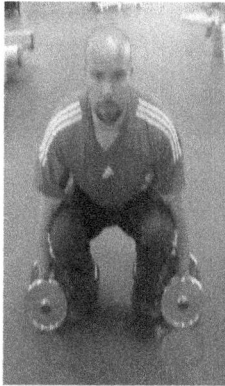
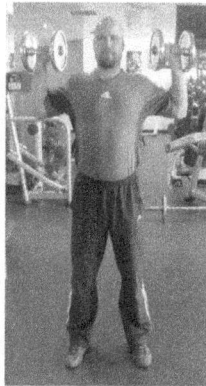

(1)   (2)

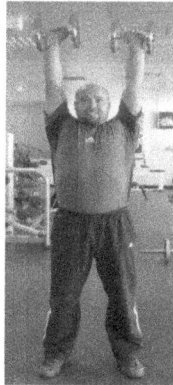

(3)

C: Stand up & raise the dumbbells to your shoulders & then above your head whilst breathing out. Attempt to do this at speed whilst using your abs

Stretching your abdominals

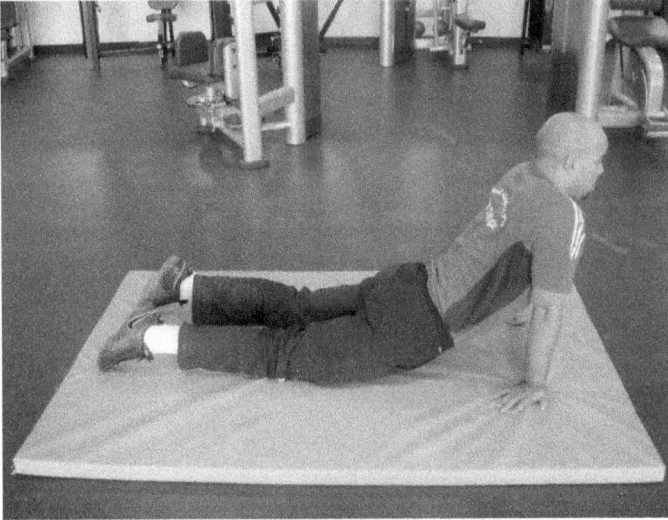

Lie on your front with your hips as close to the floor as possible, lift your upper body from the floor using your arms and push your hips into the floor. Breathe normally throughout the stretch without holding your breath.

To stretch your obliques, quite simply lie on a fit-ball (on your side) and lower your upper body below the height of your hips to ensure you get a good stretch, obviously ensure you are stable and your bottom leg is firmly on the ground.

Abdominal program – (template)

Abdominal exercises can be done as active rest for e.g. between your strength exercise sets, as a separate workout or can even be used to compliment your session i.e. completed at the end of your workout. When using weights you must ensure that your safety comes first, make sure that your technique is perfected before you increase the weight.

BEGINNER EXERCISES	REPS 10-100+	SETS 1-10	REMARKS (weight)
Bent knee Sit Up			
(Exercise A)			
(Exercise B)			
Leg Raises			
(Exercise A)			
(Exercise B)			
(Exercise C)			
(Exercise D)			
(Exercise E)			
Sit Ups (arms above head)			
(Exercise A)			
(Exercise B)			
(Exercise C)			
Sit Ups (hands on head)			
(Exercise A)			
(Exercise B)			
(Exercise C)			
Utilising a fit-ball			
(Exercise A)			
(Exercise B)			
(Exercise C)			
(Exercise D)			
Beginner Machines			
(Exercise A)			
(Exercise B)			
(Exercise C)			
INTERMEDIATE EXERCISES	**REPS**	**SETS**	**REMARKS**
Weighted ball in hands			

163

(Exercise A)			
(Exercise B)			
(Exercise C)			
(Exercise D)			
Weighted ball in feet			
(Exercise A)			
(Exercise B)			
(Exercise C)			
Partner Exercises			
(Exercise A)			
(Exercise B)			
(Exercise C)			
(Exercise D)			
Utilising a fit-ball			
(Exercise A)			
(Exercise B)			
(Exercise C)			
(Exercise D)			
ADVANCED EXERCISES	**REPS**	**SETS**	**REMARKS** (weight)
B/wt & minimum equipment			
(Exercise A)			
(Exercise B)			
(Exercise C)			
Utilising machines			
(Exercise A)			
(Exercise B)			
(Exercise C)			
Utilising barbell			
(Exercise A)			
(Exercise B)			
(Exercise C)			
(Exercise D)			
(Exercise A)			
(Exercise F)			
Utilising dumbbells			
(Exercise A)			
(Exercise B)			
(Exercise C)			

Chapter 7: Planning your workout

Whole body workshop have included templates and specific programs for you, however before jumping straight on in there, you need to know about certain considerations that you should take into account before commencing your workout.

First and foremost you should select which program is best for you i.e. what is your aim?

Aim:
- a) To Improve your flexibility;
- b) To strengthen and tone your body;
- c) To improve your muscle endurance, power or strength;
- d) To improve your muscle mass;
- e) To lose weight or
- f) Anything else...

Once you have decided on your aim, you can then move forwards with your plan:

Plan your workout routine - i.e. when can you realistically train and how often?

Below are routine examples:

TRAINING DAYS (W)	MON	TUES	WEDS	THURS	FRI	SAT	SUN
2 days a wk	W	Off	Off	W	Off	Off	Off
3 days a wk	W	Off	W	Off	W	Off	Off
4 days a wk	W	Off	W	Off	W	Off	W
Every 3 days	W	Off	Off	W	Off	Off	W

Other circumstances will be important for you to deal with such as family, friends, workout timings and location, to name but a few. Your goals, level of motivation and the way you stick to your plan will be the deciding factors for better results. Replacing negative thoughts with positive ones, having realistic goals (food choices and exercise) and visualising what you want to look or feel like are all contributing factors to success. Writing in a workout diary, why you want something (in the positive context) i.e. I want to look toned so I can look good on the beach (instead of, so I don't look fat). Write down everything you do i.e. how you felt on a particular day, why you didn't like a particular exercise and why you got better results doing a set routine more so than another. Being positive about your new routine and how you can tailor it to your needs, desires and personal goals will ensure that you become more motivated through your new way of thinking.

Your time constraints will dictate what your program will include and of course the length of each workout will be specific to your needs. If your belief is that each workout should take 40 minutes (inclusive of warm up) then for some this can be realistic, although some sessions should take longer and will ultimately depend on implementing rest periods between sets, amongst other things.

There are many books out there that will be attractive to individuals who want quick results due to busy lifestyles. These books advertise shorter workouts, quicker and better results, and the fact is that if you are proficient at exercising related to technique and safety etc and your time is limited then you can exercise in 2 minutes flat and feel better that you have done something – it's purely a psychological battle and if you have the time then you may as well use it in a safe and effective manner.

Remember, your aim will always dictate the length of time you should spend exercising and of course your personal desires about your body will dictate the level of effort i.e. the intensity of each workout you do. For example if you are on vacation and your partner is in the shower and you feel the need to push out some sit ups, push-ups and squats then you do this because time is limited, you are on holiday and you know you will feel better after doing (as good as) a whole body workout in a confined space in a minimum amount of time.

The most relevant words and abbreviations that are used throughout this book are shown below. If you are a complete beginner you may not understand some of them:

167

- **Reps** = The act of performing an exercise again;
- **Sets** = Several exercises intended to be done in series;
- **Glutes** = Gluteus muscles;
- **Add** = Adductor muscles and
- **Abd** = Abductor muscles.

On the following pages we have included a few program examples for you.

2 DAY WORKOUT – Muscle Toning

Day 1 (for e.g. Monday)

BODY PART & EXERCISES	MUSCLE ENDURANCE 13-20 Reps	SETS 1-3	RECOVERY (Minutes)
Leg exercises	Reps	Sets	Rest
Static Hold	20	1	2
Bridge	20	1	2
Squat	20	1	2
Chest exercises	Reps	Sets	Rest
Isometric hold	20	1	2
Incline Push Ups	20	1	2
Normal Push Ups	20	1	2
Back exercises	Reps	Sets	Rest
Back extensions	20	1	2
Alt arm/leg raise 1	20	1	2
Shoulder exercises	Reps	Sets	Rest
Isometric holds 1-4	20	1	2
Advanced Hold	20	1	2
Bicep exercises	Reps	Sets	Rest
Isometric hold	20	1	2
Partner Res Holds	20	1	2
Triceps exercises	Reps	Sets	Rest
Bench Dips	20	1	2
Incline Press Ups	20	1	2
Advanced press ups	20	1	2

Refer to pages 42-74 for descriptions of all bodyweight exercises

Day 2 (for e.g. Wednesday)

BODY PART & EXERCISES	MUSCLE ENDURANCE 13-20 REPS	SETS 1-3	RECOVERY (Minutes)
Leg exercises	Reps	Sets	Rest
Lunge	15	2	1
Step Up	15	2	1
Squat Jump	15	2	1
Chest exercises	Reps	Sets	Rest
Decline Push Ups	15	2	1
Bodyweight Dips	15	2	1
Back exercises	Reps	Sets	Rest
Straight leg hold	15	2	1
Plank progressions	15	2	1
Shoulder Exercises	Reps	Sets	Rest
Partner Resisted Ex's	15	2	1
Caterpillar	15	2	1
Additional Holds	15	2	1
Bicep exercises	Reps	Sets	Rest
Under-grasp pull ups	15	2	1
Behind neck pull ups	15	2	1
Triceps exercises	Reps	Sets	Rest
Partner walk	15	2	1
Body raises	15	2	1

Remarks

The above programs are examples for working muscle endurance. When you are confident enough to increase the sets from 1-2 or 2-3 then you can decrease the rest time accordingly from 2 minutes to 1 minute. You can also alter your reps to compensate for completing more sets (as shown in the above program). These programs are not set in stone and you should progress according to your own personal fitness level i.e. once you have mastered the technique and you feel competent enough, increase the sets and adjust the reps and rest intervals accordingly.

Refer to pages 42-74 for descriptions of all bodyweight exercises

3 DAY WORKOUT – Muscle Toning

Day 1 (for e.g. Monday)

BODY PART & EXERCISES	MUSCLE ENDURANCE 13-20 REPS	SETS 1-4	RECOVERY (Minutes)
Shoulder exercises	Reps	Sets	Rest
Isometric holds 1-4	15	3-4	1-2
Advanced Hold	15	3-4	1-2
Partner Resisted Ex's	15	3-4	1-2
Caterpillar	15	3-4	1-2
Additional Holds	15	3-4	1-2
Leg exercises	Reps	Sets	Rest
Static Hold	15	3-4	1-2
Bridge	15	3-4	1-2
Squat	15	3-4	1-2
Lunge	15	3-4	1-2
Step Up	15	3-4	1-2
Squat Jump	15	3-4	1-2

Day 2 (for e.g. Wednesday)

BODY PART & EXERCISES	MUSCLE ENDURANCE 13-20 REPS	SETS 1-4	RECOVERY (Minutes)
Back exercises	Reps	Sets	Rest
Back extensions	15	3-4	1-2
Alt arm/leg raise 1&2	15	3-4	1-2
Straight leg hold	15	3-4	1-2
Plank progressions	15	3-4	1-2
Hip raises	15	3-4	1-2
Bicep exercises	Reps	Sets	Rest
Isometric hold	15	3-4	1-2
Partner Res Holds	15	3-4	1-2
Under-grasp pull ups	15	3-4	1-2
Behind neck pull ups	15	3-4	1-2

Day 3 (for e.g. Friday)

BODY PART & EXERCISES	MUSCLE ENDURANCE 13-20 REPS	SETS 1-4	RECOVERY (Minutes)
Chest exercises	Reps	Sets	Rest
Isometric hold	15	3-4	1-2
Incline Push Ups	15	3-4	1-2
Normal Push Ups	15	3-4	1-2
Decline Push Ups	15	3-4	1-2
Bodyweight Dips	15	3-4	1-2
Triceps exercises	Reps	Sets	Rest
Bench Dips	15	3-4	1-2
Incline Press Ups	15	3-4	1-2
Advanced press ups	15	3-4	1-2
Partner walk	15	3-4	1-2
Body raises	15	3-4	1-2

Remarks

Adequate rest should be taken between each set i.e. (1 or 2 minutes) so ensure that you are fully recovered prior to commencing the next exercise or quite simply exercise another body part as part of active rest i.e. with the examples above you can alternate the 2 body parts to ensure adequate rest. It is advised that a day of rest (complete or active rest) should be taken between each day of strength training and if you choose active rest then this could include doing some cardio, working on your abdominals or simply stretching.

Refer to pages 42-74 for descriptions of all bodyweight exercises.

4 DAY RESISTANCE BAND WORKOUT -
Muscle strength

Colour band used (_____)

Day 1

BODY PART & EXERCISES	MUSCLE STRENGTH 6-12 REPS	SETS 1-4	RECOVERY (Minutes)
Back exercises	Reps	Sets	Rest
Bent over row	8	3-4	2-3
Chest exercises	Reps	Sets	Rest
Flyes 1	8	3-4	2-3
Shoulder exercises	Reps	Sets	Rest
Shoulder Press	8	3-4	2-3
Bicep exercises	Reps	Sets	Rest
Standing Curls	8	3-4	2-3
Triceps exercises	Reps	Sets	Rest
Overhead press	8	3-4	2-3
Leg exercises	Reps	Sets	Rest
Squats	8	3-4	2-3

Day 2

BODY PART & EXERCISES	MUSCLE STRENGTH 6-12 REPS	SETS 1-4	RECOVERY (Minutes)
Back exercises	Reps	Sets	Rest
Seated row	8	3-4	2-3
Chest exercises	Reps	Sets	Rest
Chest Press	8	3-4	2-3
Shoulder exercises	Reps	Sets	Rest
Frontal Raise	8	3-4	2-3
Bicep exercises	Reps	Sets	Rest
Overhead Pull	8	3-4	2-3
Triceps exercises	Reps	Sets	Rest
Kickbacks	8	3-4	2-3
Leg exercises	Reps	Sets	Rest
Hip extension	8	3-4	2-3

Day 3

BODY PART & EXERCISES	MUSCLE STRENGTH 6-12 REPS	SETS 1-4	RECOVERY (Minutes)
Back exercises	Reps	Sets	Rest
Lat pull down	8	3-4	2-3
Chest exercises	Reps	Sets	Rest
Pullovers	8	3-4	2-3
Shoulder exercises	Reps	Sets	Rest
Lateral Raise	8	3-4	2-3
Bicep exercises	Reps	Sets	Rest
Bent over curl	8	3-4	2-3
Triceps exercises	Reps	Sets	Rest
Overhead push	8	3-4	2-3
Leg exercises	Reps	Sets	Rest
Hip flexion	8	3-4	2-3

Day 4

BODY PART & EXERCISES	MUSCLE STRENGTH 6-12 REPS	SETS 1-4	RECOVERY (Minutes)
Back exercises	Reps	Sets	Rest
Single arm row	8	3-4	2-3
Chest exercises	Reps	Sets	Rest
Flyes 2 or 3	8	3-4	2-3
Shoulder exercises	Reps	Sets	Rest
Isometric Holds	8	3-4	2-3
Bicep exercises	Reps	Sets	Rest
Isometric Hold	8	3-4	2-3
Triceps exercises	Reps	Sets	Rest
Forward press	8	3-4	2-3
Leg exercises	Reps	Sets	Rest
Abd & Adduction	8	3-4	2-3

Remarks

When you are ready, increase the amount of reps per exercise and lower the rest intervals to ensure you work harder for longer periods. These programs are examples only and how you plan your workout is entirely up to you and dependant on many factors i.e. how much time you have, how quickly you are learning the technique of each exercise and other factors already covered in this book.

Refer to pages 76-102 for descriptions of all resistance band exercises

Summary

As with every exercise workout, you can make it as easy or as difficult as you choose and this book was put together in such a way that the exercises shown are progressive according to your present fitness level. You can of course begin where you feel more comfortable so long as you are safe. Of course there are many more exercises you can do for your whole body but this selection contains specific groups of exercises which utilise your own bodyweight, the fit-ball and other equipment to further ensure that your whole body is worked thoroughly. The selected exercises complement each other and with the respective progressions you can definitely challenge yourself accordingly and get enormous benefit from using them in a correct and safe manner. Ensure as always that you warm up and stretch accordingly prior to any exercise and more importantly cool down and stretch for longer on completion of your workout in order to prevent injuries and reduce muscle soreness.

Utilising equipment such as the fit-ball and weighted balls etc prevent you from repetition of the same bodyweight exercises and will ultimately add variety to your training. If you use the fit-ball to compliment your normal routine then it is advised that you complete them towards the latter part of your workout. Focus is the key factor with core strength training which in turn ensures that your body remains balanced, not just on the fit-ball but with reference to its musculature and respective supporting structures. Training with weights is the most beneficial and most under-rated way to work your whole body especially with regards to weight loss. So many people think that you need to do just sit ups to work the abs, but the exercises with weights if done correctly and safely require a large amount of strength from your abdominals and this is due to the majority of your power coming from this area.

Safety is the key factor, so long as you master the technique with minimum resistance/weight initially and progress accordingly. Muscle imbalances can and will cause problems in other areas of your body, especially later in life. These imbalances should be looked at immediately by tightening and stretching the relevant muscles involved explained in more detail within visualise the 'new you' book & the rehabilitation

176

books on the website below, maintaining good posture at all times will undoubtedly help too. The amount of repetitions and sets you do will depend on your current level of fitness, try out all of the exercises and create a program for yourself using the templates provided. Depending on your aim and how you plan your time and workout program, your personal success will only be dictated by you.

Whole body workshop can only provide the information; you must provide the mind and body to complement the content.

Edition 2 will be waiting for you once you reach a plateau and only you will know when the time is right to advance on the knowledge and success you will possess after utilising what 'Exercise your whole body at home' has provided for you. More info on types of programs etc can be found on the website:

www.wholebodyworkshop.com
info@wholebodyworkshop.com